Health Service Quality

An introduction to quality methods for Health Services

JOHN ØVRETVEIT

Professor of Health
Organisation and Management
The Nordic School of Public Health
Göteborg, Sweden

FOREWORD BY
CHRISTINA TOWNSEND
NHS Training Director

**Blackwell
Science**

UCSM

© 1992 by
Blackwell Science Ltd
Editorial Offices:
Osney Mead, Oxford OX2 0EL
25 John Street, London WC1N 2BL
23 Ainslie Place, Edinburgh EH3 6AJ
238 Main Street, Cambridge
  Massachusetts 02142, USA
54 University Street, Carlton
  Victoria 3053, Australia

Other Editorial Offices:
Arnette Blackwell SA
  224, Boulevard Saint Germain
  75007 Paris, France

Blackwell Wissenschafts-Verlag GmbH
  Kurfürstendamm 57
  10707 Berlin, Germany

  Zehetnergasse 6
  A-1140 Wien
  Austria

First published 1992
Reprinted 1992, 1994, 1995, 1996

Set by Setrite Typesetters, Hong Kong
Printed and bound in Great Britain
at the University Press, Cambridge

The Blackwell Science logo is a
trade mark of Blackwell Science Ltd,
registered at the United Kingdom
Trade Marks Registry

DISTRIBUTORS

  Marston Book Services Ltd
  PO Box 269
  Abingdon
  Oxon OX14 4YN
  (Orders: Tel: 01235 465500
          Fax: 01235 465555)

USA
  Blackwell Science, Inc.
  238 Main Street
  Cambridge, MA 02142
  (Orders: Tel: 800 215-1000
          617 876-7000
          Fax: 617 492-5263)

Canada
  Copp Clark, Ltd
  2775 Matheson Blvd East
  Mississauga, Ontario
  Canada, L4W 4P7
  (Orders: Tel: 800 263-4374
          905 238-6074

Australia
  Blackwell Science Pty Ltd
  54 University Street
  Carlton, Victoria 3053
  (Orders: Tel: 03 9347 0300
          Fax: 03 9347 5001)

British Library
Cataloguing in Publication Data
Øvretveit, John
  Health service quality
  I. Title
  362.10685

ISBN 0-632-03279-0

Contents

Appendices 163

Foreword

ACHIEVING QUALITY health services depends as much on people as it does on systems and techniques. As the author makes clear in his preface, the recognition of this fact is a major reason for writing this book. In particular, he is concerned there is a danger that the new systems for standard-setting and inspection will be adopted readily while the necessary attitudes, skills and working relationships go largely ignored and undeveloped.

Nowhere is this more relevant than in the NHS, which is both a very people-intensive organization and one in which team working is essential. As the NHS Training Director, I welcome this book not only because it emphasizes people, skills and working relationships, but also because it shows how NHS staff can begin to use and adapt quality tools to improve services and achieve health gain.

Dr Christina Townsend
NHS Training Director

THE 1990s WILL SEE a crisis in health. Many countries are facing similar problems in trying to meet rising demand with fewer health care workers, contain rising costs, and yet ensure that there is choice and that providers are responsive to individuals' needs. Never has so much been possible with so few resources.

It is becoming clearer that part of the solution must be new political processes for deciding how to allocate resources (e.g. the Oregon experiment in the USA (*BMJ* 1991)). Many European countries view regulated markets as part of the solution. However, I believe that it will be quality methods and philosophies, adapted to the special circumstances of health services, that will emerge as the most important response to the problems of health provision in the 1990s.

This book introduces quality methods and outlines an approach to quality developed for health services. Although it is written primarily for people who work in the British NHS, the concepts and ideas are also relevant to private health services and health systems in Europe, the USA, Australia and other countries.

In Britain, the 1990 government NHS reforms put quality on the agenda for the first time (DoH 1989). Providers wondered how to establish professional audit, and how to demonstrate the quality of their service to purchasers, and in some cases to referrers and clients as well. Purchasers wanted to specify quality in contracts, as well as price and quantity. Some were sceptical as to whether the NHS reforms would improve services, but felt that the risks would be reduced if purchasers were concerned about quality. There was also some evidence that providers would compete on quality, at least as much as on price. But given the many changes and deadlines it was not surprising that quality was viewed as yet another requirement imposed by the reforms, and with the same enthusiasm as many of the other changes.

Few recognized that quality is not a purchaser requirement to be met, but a philosophy, a set of methods, and an organizational revolution essential to the competitive position and survival of a service; that quality improves customer service, cuts costs and raises productivity. Fewer still recognized that continuous quality improvement must be driven by the service provider, not the purchaser. Those that did recognize this, and were aware of the experiences of manufacturing and commercial services in this field, were daunted by the magnitude of the task of introducing a quality approach into a health service.

One reason for writing this book was because I felt that the quality approach was in danger of being misunderstood and misapplied in the NHS, and of becoming discredited with staff. My concern is that the quality approach could be undermined in the NHS and in other health services by a bureaucratic culture. This is a culture that readily adopts inspection and standard-setting imposed from above, a culture that ignores the revolution in human relations and attitudes that is as much a part of the quality approach as the techniques, disciplines and systems.

I argue that, even if health services begin to use the new quality tools and techniques which I describe, there will be little sustained improvement unless there are also fundamental changes in the way people think about and do their work. Quality is as much about changing the way people relate to each other and about making working life more satisfying as it is about systems and standard-setting.

Another theme of the book is the need to take a comprehensive and systematic view to realize the full value of the quality approach, whatever the size of the service unit. This involves using simple techniques first and building up a quality system, as well as ensuring a balance between the three dimensions of quality: Client, Professional and Management Quality.

This book is mainly for practitioners, managers and other health service staff who are interested in using quality approaches. It shows how they can adapt and apply these approaches to improve the quality of their service. It draws on consultancy research into quality in commercial services that convinced me that quality approaches could help with many of the current problems in health services.

More recently the climate was right to begin to apply and develop these ideas with staff in the British NHS. The results of that work are reported here. The framework provides a systematic and comprehensive approach for linking business strategy to a quality system, and a framework within which to apply the methods.

In order to help the reader, certain parts of the text appear within boxes: grey tinted boxes in the text and margin are summaries or examples, while blue tinted boxes highlight central concepts and definitions.

Acknowledge-ments

M Y THANKS TO the Brunel Institute and to the managers and practitioners with whom I worked for making possible the research which is reported here. Few research institutes in the UK could have provided me with the experience of working with managers and staff on quality issues in so many different public and private services, and provided the interdisciplinary environment in which to develop the ideas. My thanks in particular to Alan Dale of the Programme for Service, and to Anna, Rick, Mary, and Marie.

I would also like to thank Glaxo Pharmaceuticals UK Ltd for sponsoring the publication of this book and for helping to make it available to a wide readership within the British NHS and in other health services.

1

Introduction and Overview

WE OFTEN THINK of a quality service as one which gives us what we want — that quality is customer satisfaction. Quality in this book means something different. It means a service which gives people what they need, as well as what they want, and does so at the lowest cost.

Health services face increasing problems in achieving these sometimes conflicting aims. More health services are finding that they can only do so by making use of a set of proven methods and a philosophy — termed here 'the quality approach'. This book describes these ideas and shows how they can be applied in health services.

This chapter is a general introduction to 'the quality approach'. It aims to convey a flavour of the quality philosophy and of the key principles of the approach. It also introduces a framework which was developed and applied in different health services and which recognizes the culture and circumstances of these services. This introduction is by way of answers to five common questions raised by people when they first consider quality. The chapter finishes with an overview of the book.

What I term the 'quality approach' is a body of knowledge and experience developed over the last 60 years in a variety of organizations. As in many disciplines there is no single unified theory, but a number of approaches, some more theoretically based than others. All emphasize a systematic and scientific approach to organizational improvement and the need to train and encourage all employees to use simple methods to improve their working processes. Some of the most exciting recent developments in the field have come from the use of quality methods in service industries. It is only in the last few years that quality methods have been applied in health services.

If I had to sum up the book in a sentence it would be that people and perfect processes make a quality health service. A poor quality service results from a badly designed and operated process, not from lazy or incompetent health workers. Continual quality improvement comes from giving people the new methods and skills to analyse quality problems and processes, and by empowering them to make the necessary changes. It does not come from inspection and standard-setting, nor simply from exhortation and customer relations training.

> **Quality: five common questions**
> - What is 'the quality approach'?
> - What is quality in health services?
> - What are the features of a 'quality approach'?
> - How can a quality approach help with some of the current problems in health services?
> - What are the different approaches to quality, and which are most relevant to a particular type of health service?

What is 'the quality approach'?

Generally 'quality' is an umbrella term for a coordinated set of staff and organizational development activities. It builds on existing strengths and good practices, but it is different from other development programmes in that it enables staff to use new methods in a systematic way to control quality and to resolve quality problems.

Successful quality programmes pay as much attention to changing human relations — relations between managers and staff and staff and patients — as to introducing new systems, and to specification and measurement. There needs to be as much emphasis on changing people's attitude towards their work as on training them to use specific tools and methods. Tools are only used if people want to use them. They are only used properly if people have been trained to use them and have the time to do so.

Successful programmes lay as much emphasis on recognizing existing good practice and standards as on developing new standards and procedures, but again, only in the full understanding of the purpose of specification. A systematic approach is essential, but so is the belief in and understanding of why these approaches are being used. Unsuccessful programmes produce either systems without spirit, or passion without perfect processes.

What is quality in health services?

In this book quality in health services is defined as:

> 'Fully meeting requirements at the lowest cost,'
> or, more specifically,
> 'Fully meeting the needs of those who need the service most, at the lowest cost to the organization, within limits and directives set by higher authorities and purchasers'

This definition of quality is different from many others. For example, there are definitions of quality in terms of:

Features of service. For example, accessibility, relevance to need, equity, social acceptability, efficiency and effectiveness (Maxwell 1984). But this misses an idea which is central to the quality approach: the idea of customer responsiveness and of giving customers what they want. How do we know that customers put these features first? Research suggests that they value other features (Parasuraman *et al.* 1985, 1988; discussed in Chapter 3). Another definition of quality is in terms of:

2

Customer satisfaction. For example, 'fully meeting customer requirements', or 'The totality of features and characteristics of a product or service that bear on its ability to satisfy stated or implied needs' (BSI 1990). In health services, quality is sometimes seen only as improving customer satisfaction.

Whilst this is one aspect of quality, it is important not just to produce satisfaction for those clients or patients (here-after termed 'clients') who receive the service, but to ensure that all who need the service can and do get it, especially in public health services. This responsibility for others apart from those in contact involves assessing population needs and targeting — implied in my definition by *'meeting the needs of those who need the service most'*.

Chapter 2 considers the responsibilities of agencies which purchase health services (e.g. in England and Wales, District Health Authorities (DHAs)) and of providers in these respects. It is the responsibility of purchasing authorities to assess the health needs of populations and to place contracts with providers for certain services to meet needs. Providers have to show that their services get to those most in need and to show that they prioritize within different client groups. The point here is that one dimension of quality is what those in contact with a service think about it *and* whether the service gets to those most in need.

However, we cannot define quality only in terms of client satisfaction and expressed demand. The clients of health services may not know what they need, or may ask for treatments that really are inappropriate or harmful. We have to include alongside the client's judgement of the service a professional definition of need, and a professional judgement of the extent to which a service meets the client's needs.

These points are implicit in my deliberate use of the ambiguous term 'need'. This recognizes that need is defined by clients and by professionals, at an individual level and at a population level. 'Professionals' means professional service providers as well as external referrers such as General Medical Practitioners.

Quality is meeting needs. A service, then, may meet customers' needs, as perceived by them and by professionals, and be effective. But a service that did this still might not be a quality service. It may be inefficient and wasteful of resources — resources that could be used to treat more clients.

A quality service is not one that meets customers' needs at any cost (the quickest way of going out of business) but one that uses its resources in the most efficient way. Hence the element of my definition *'meeting needs at the lowest cost'*, the lowest cost usually being the lowest cost compared to competitors.

Finally a service could not be high quality if it did not meet legal, ethical, contractual and other 'higher level' requirements — hence *'within limits and directives set by higher authorities/purchasers'* in the definition.

In summary, the definition recognizes that a quality health service is one that satisfies a number of sometimes conflicting requirements and interest groups. Health service quality involves three dimensions: Client, Professional and Management Quality.

The three dimensions of health service quality

Client Quality:
What clients and carers want from the service
(individuals and populations)
Professional Quality:
Whether the service meets needs as defined by
professional providers and referrers, and whether it
correctly carries out techniques and procedures which are
believed to be necessary to meet client needs
Management Quality:
The most efficient and productive use of resources,
within limits and directives set by higher authorities/
purchasers

These dimensions correspond to the major interest groups whose perspectives must be integrated to specify the quality of a particular service. That is, the interests of clients, carers (where relevant), referrers (mostly GPs), professional providers, management, and purchasers (mostly health authorities and budget-holding GPs). This complexity is one of the differences between health services and many other services.

How does the 'quality approach' help with the difficulty of satisfying all of these interests? How can a provider achieve high Client, Professional and Management Quality all at the same time? The rest of this book could be considered an answer to this question, but we need to pause here to give two answers.

It is not possible to achieve quality without defining what it means. The above concept of quality directs us towards defining standards of quality for each dimension. Because standards define precisely what a service has to provide, having standards clarifies exactly where there are conflicts. This makes it possible to face up to conflicts with explicit statements and trade-offs.

For example, health and safety and fire regulations may require certain standards which conflict with patients' preferences and professional standards of care. Setting standards

4

helps to be more precise about the conflict which makes it easier to work out solutions, especially by involving the different parties.

Quality methods also direct towards making changes that, at the same time, improve quality from all perspectives. An example is methods for analysing the service as a process (explained in Chapter 3). A process analysis may identify lost patient records as a quality problem. Quality methods can then be used to seek out and remove the causes of this problem using a Quality Correction Cycle (Chapter 5). Avoiding lost patient records thus contributes to raising the Professional Quality of the service, reducing costs (raising the Management Quality), and to fewer delays for the client (raising the Client Quality).

The 'quality approach' is not magic as some suggest, but a set of methods and a philosophy. The approach to quality described in this book forces people to face up to the conflicts of interest, to situations where raising one aspect of quality inevitably lowers another, and to work out explicit resolutions to such conflicts. The methods focus attention on making changes which have multiple benefits.

What are the features of a 'quality approach'?

Quality terms are often confusing to newcomers to the subject, not least because they are used in different ways by different people (Appendix 1 gives a Glossary of Terms). Before looking at the relevance of quality methods and concepts to health services, more needs to be said about what the methods and concepts are and how they fit together. The following also shows the sequence in which they should be introduced to a service.

Set standards. The starting point is to define quality for a particular service as a set of quality standards. This defines the key features of quality on the three dimensions of Client, Professional and Management Quality. The decision about which standards to set and how to set them is critical. Chapter 6 considers sources and criteria for selecting standards.

Chapter 2 discusses how business strategy should influence the selection of quality standards. Chapters 3, 4 and 5 discuss how to set standards and measure performance from the Client, Professional and Management Quality perspectives respectively.

Measure performance. Once quality is defined as standards, then the quality of the service can be measured. Different methods are used to measure and document what is happening and to compare this against what is intended. The principle is to select a few standards to measure routinely, and to have a broader set for annual reviews.

Take action. This may be either congratulatory or corrective. Where quality performance is poor, a subject is picked for corrective action. Quality methods are used to select which subject to focus on (e.g. quality costing methods (Chapter 5)), to involve staff in gathering ideas about causes ('fish-bone' diagrams and quality groups (Chapter 5)), to collect data about possible causes of problems (chart and graph methods), to decide what changes to make and to evaluate the results. This is the 'Quality Correction Cycle' which finishes when the cause of the quality problem is removed.

Repeat the 'Quality Management Cycle'. The idea of the Quality Management Cycle is to ensure that staff in a service carry out each of the steps above. Sometimes a service gets stuck at the standard-setting stage — there are too many standards to measure, even annually. Sometimes a service does measure and document quality performance, but does not take any action. Sometimes all the steps are carried out but the service does not periodically revise its standards.

Establish a quality system. One of the reasons services do not carry out the Quality Management Cycle is that they do not have a quality system. A quality system is the roles, responsibilities, processes and procedures which an organization has to ensure that staff are able to, and do, carry out quality management. One of the aims of a quality system is to improve the way quality is improved: to review how well the Quality Management Cycle is being carried out and to make changes to make it work better (e.g. more training).

The assumption is that the cost of a quality system is more than offset by the savings. In some sectors, purchasers will only consider contracting providers who have a quality system (see Chapter 7). Some approaches to *accreditation* assess the quality system of a service (e.g. BSI 5750), whereas others assess the past performance of the service against a set of quality standards.

Review professional audit. The main way in which quality is currently improved in health services is by each professional group carrying out audit. There are advantages to starting in this way (Chapter 4), but sooner or later these approaches will need to be modified. This is because (a) the most pressing quality problems are due to poor cooperation between professions, (b) many health services are provided through multidisciplinary teams and need multidisciplinary solutions, and (c) traditional audit concentrates on Professional Quality issues and ignores the Client Quality and Management Quality dimensions. Chapter 4 considers whether to broaden existing audit, or to integrate different professions' approaches.

Develop quality assurance. A service carrying out the Quality Management Cycle is undertaking quality assurance. A quality system ensures that this is done. In time, a service will be able to focus more on predicting and preventing quality problems, and will use more sophisticated quality methods to prevent and predict poor quality (e.g. statistical process control (Chapter 6)).

Introduce total quality management. When staff have been trained and have experience in using quality methods, and when they are familiar with the Quality Management Cycle, it is possible to consider introducing Total Quality Management (TQM). This takes the quality approach a step further and aims to ensure that all staff practise the methods and philosophy of quality. Some quality strategies fail because this step is taken too early. It is impossible to introduce TQM without a quality system, and this takes some time to establish.

At the end of this chapter there is an overview of the book, showing where these ideas are discussed in more detail. With this short introduction to quality terms we can now return to the relevance of these ideas to health services.

How can a quality approach help with some of the current problems in health services?

Across the western world both demand for and costs of health services are rising. The problems that result are especially acute in public health services. In a publicly financed health service, demand will always be greater than supply and resources, irrespective of demographics and medical technology. Political solutions to rationing are necessary, but so are solutions in the improved provision of services. Adapting and developing quality methods in health services is one of the main ways of meeting the challenges facing health services in the 1990s. However, at a time when services are under more pressure than ever it is extremely difficult to find development finance to invest in a quality programme, and for managers and staff to give the extra time and energy which is needed to apply these methods.

In the past, if a public service did raise quality, then demand went up and put extra pressure on fixed resources, which in turn led to a drop in quality. There was therefore no incentive to raise quality. In the private sector the whole point of improving quality is to increase or maintain demand in order to make profit. In public services there was not the link between increased demand, higher profits, growth and material incentives for staff.

In the UK the 1990 NHS reforms may change this, but even without the reforms there are other reasons for adopting a quality approach:

1 *Raising the Management Quality of the service reduces the cost of poor quality and frees resources*, usually quite dramatically in the early stages. The general estimate is that between 30 and 50% of operating costs can be saved by resolving internal quality problems (Chapter 5).

2 *Work is easier, less frustrating and more satisfying for staff*. This is especially so if staff devise and carry out improvements, which gives them further incentives to raise quality (Chapter 8). Staff want to work in a quality service, and this makes recruitment and retention easier. Many improvements usually also make it possible for the service to respond to clients more quickly.

3 *Defuses dissatisfaction by negotiating expectations*. Attention to Client Quality means making clear what service can be provided with the resources. One way to avoid client dissatisfaction is to manage expectations (Chapter 3). This involves explaining to a client the rationing criteria and constraints, and negotiating what can be done. At the level of the population it means involving the public in deciding the rationing criteria (e.g. the Oregon experiment in the USA (*BMJ* 1991)).

4 *Avoids negligence claims*. Compensation awards alone are approaching 1% of UK health authority budgets and are set to rise dramatically. In the UK the change to provider units paying for negligence claims awarded against them will begin to have an impact from 1993 onwards. Many claims would not become formal claims if attention were paid to Client Quality, regardless of whether or not there was negligence or error. Most people only want an apology, or an assurance that the same thing will not happen to someone else.

5 *Bad reputation means lost income if there is choice*. As soon as people have a choice of service other costs become relevant. Suppose 1% of clients are so dissatisfied that they are moved to make a formal complaint. Research into other services shows that a reasonable estimate is that at least

10% of clients do not complain but go elsewhere (TARP 1980). On average each one of these 10% tells 10 other people of their dissatisfaction (13% tell over 20) and these other people will be inclined to go elsewhere. In the UK they will tell their referring GP of their preference. If the GP is a budget holder they will be influenced by the patient's view to refer elsewhere (Fig. 1.1).

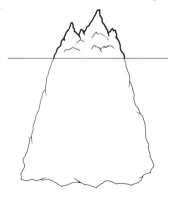

1% of clients make a formal complaint (potential negligence claim)

10% don't complain but go elsewhere (Lost income. Difficult to win clients back)

Each of the 10% tells others of their dissatisfaction. Others prefer to go elsewhere. More lost income. Bad reputation takes years to overcome.

Fig. 1.1 Formal complaints are the tip of the iceberg of dissatisfaction.

The implications are that if there are alternatives, a service which sets 1% formal complaints as an acceptable level will not survive. Although investing in quality costs money, this cost has to be set against both the potential lost income and the current cost of internal poor quality.

6 *Values professional staff and improves interprofessional cooperation.* Another reason for adopting a quality approach is that attention to Professional Quality, for example in professional audit, recognizes the importance of professional staff. People want to work in a quality service, and with increasingly competitive labour markets quality is important to recruit and retain staff.

A service with high Professional Quality enhances pride in professionalism, and contributes to removing mistakes and delays. Improvements to Professional Quality also means better coordination and communications between professionals, which in turn save time and money. More will be said in Chapter 8 about the incentives for staff and managers to introduce quality and of the cost savings.

7 *Competitive advantage.* Another reason to introduce a quality approach is that the early adopters, be they a public or a private health service, will gain a competitive advantage. In time, others will not be able to compete for contracts or for good staff. Experience in other sectors shows that it is

difficult to catch up. Commercial services in finance, travel and other sectors have recognized these facts and are making massive investments in quality programmes.

> Failure to introduce quality means that the already wide gap between the service we receive in many public health services and the service we receive in the high street and other areas will widen. The public are already making comparisons and asking why they should not expect the same standards of service which are becoming common elsewhere. More are choosing private health services.

This is not to suggest that a quality approach is a magic cure-all, or that it is simple to introduce. Nor that there are not important differences between commercial and public services which need to be considered when developing an approach which is right for a particular hospital, community service or family practitioner service. Rather, I am proposing that the quality approach is not just relevant to the current problems in health services, but that it is also essential to the future of public services such as the NHS.

What are the different approaches to quality, and which are most relevant to a particular type of health service?

Most health service staff think of a quality approach as audit (e.g. medical or nursing), possibly supplemented by surveys and 'customer relations training'. In those services where a number of these different initiatives are pursued they are often not brought together or coordinated as part of a sustained strategy for quality. As a result the approach to quality is partial, there are fewer benefits for the time and energy invested, and there are many different views in teams and across the service about the purpose of quality activities.

To raise quality, and to continue to do so, a health service must have a quality framework and a strategy for introducing quality methods and for ensuring that the methods are used across the service — in short an overall 'approach' to quality.

Each quality specialist puts forward their approach as being the best and only, and I am no exception (Chapter 9). This is even more true with the established experts, who, with their wider and longer experience, perhaps have more cause to crusade theirs as the true approach.

All argue that their approach is built on hard practical experience, but is also theoretically sound; is used in a wide variety of organizations but is appropriate to all; and of course is sensitive to the culture and history of the organization and flexible enough to be adapted to the unique situation of the reader's or client's organization (Deming 1986; Crosby 1979; Juran & Gryna 1980). The most well-known approaches share similar elements but disagree over emphasis and about certain points (see Appendix 6). Many packages offered by management consultancies are variations of these 'classic' approaches. Readers will have to judge for themselves whether to adopt one of these approaches or develop their own. Rather than presenting an assessment of the different approaches, the following picks out certain differences between commercial services and public and private health services. These differences should be borne in mind when deciding which type of approach to adopt. Does a chosen quality approach recognize and respond to the following special features of health services?

1 *The demand–supply–income equation.* In the British NHS until 1991, any improvement in quality which raised demand faster than supply led to stricter rationing criteria and/or longer waiting lists, because no extra resources were available. Staff employment was not threatened by poor quality and losing clients was not a problem but a relief. In commercial services, by contrast, an increase in demand leads to higher profits and finances extra resources, making possible the growth which is essential in these sectors.

In the UK it is not yet clear whether the 1990 NHS reforms will reduce the financial disincentives to raising quality in public health services. The intention is that a service which attracts more clients will get more finance. Much will depend on how purchasing health authorities set the cost–quantity–quality balance in contracts, how much they are prepared to pay to retain certain services locally, and how referring GPs act.

The reforms may not reduce the difference between the private and public sector to the extent that the same substantial investment in quality is necessary to survival. The reforms do require providers to demonstrate their quality to purchasers, but this is not a quality strategy driven by the knowledge that the service will not be there in two years if the strategy is not successful.

This difference may be summed up by saying that the health sector was not, and will not be, a free market with the same competitive pressures which stimulate quality programmes in other sectors.

2 *Availability of alternatives and attitude of clients.* Private sector clients are choosy, critical and vocal. It is easier for private services to get feedback, where the client pays for a service directly and can judge value for money. There is also

> **Differences between health and other services which are relevant to applying a quality approach**
>
> - Infinite demand but finite resources, which come mostly from public purchasing agencies
> - Undemanding clients with low expectations and little choice
> - Complex 'customer': must satisfy purchasers, referrers, the clients and their carers, rather than just a customer-purchaser
> - The 'high intangibles' content by many health services — cannot prescribe caring
> - High professional component in health services

the motive to seek out customer views because they can usually go elsewhere.

In public health services clients do not pay directly for the service and feel that they do not have the same rights to demand a quality service or to complain. How can you criticize a service which is 'free' and where all the staff are so busy and obviously doing their best? How can you demand more caring?

In the UK there is a general respect for and sentimental attitude towards the NHS. Until recently criticism of an NHS service was as likely as criticism of the Queen. Many health service recipients are vulnerable and not in a position conducive to complaint or even to comment to staff about delays. In the eyes of a groggy weak patient, a twitch of a ward sister's mouth is taken as marking them out as 'trouble' and hints at future reprisals. The 'Dunkirk' spirit will pull them through on ward 'B' (see Appendix 7).

Not only do many service recipients feel powerless, many of them are powerless even in good health. Many are in institutions, or are not used to being asked about or articulating their views, and fear the consequences of doing so. Undemanding clients and low expectations may account for some of the decline in public health services. Overcoming the 'gratitude factor' and giving patients a voice will be central to any quality approach.

In general it is more difficult to find out what clients of health services think about the service than, for example, what people think about a package holiday or hotel service. One reason is that we form our views by making comparisons. Attitudes about a service are related to the availability of alternatives — what does it matter what we think if there is no alternative?

Again, it is not clear how far the 1990 NHS reforms will increase choice and minimize these differences between public and private services. It is clear that these differences must be considered when developing and introducing a quality programme.

3 *Satisfy a range of demands*. Purchasing agencies and most providers have to satisfy a range of demands which frequently conflict. Not only is there the direct beneficiary of the service (which this book terms 'the client'), there are also the beneficiary's 'informal' carers — relatives, friends or neighbours.

Providers also have to satisfy a referrer, who in the UK is usually a GP, and may be one with a budget and hence a 'purchaser-client'. Finally, in some instances the community at large may be the client, requiring the service to act on behalf of the community to protect its well-being. Some services do have a social control function, e.g. involuntary detention under the Mental Health Act.

Which of these demands is more important? Which perceptions of the service should the service measure, and how? They all affect income in different ways so should all views be sought? How should the service resolve conflicts resulting from trying to satisfy all these demands? How far can a service target a particular client group, or must it be 'open-door'?

Answers to these questions are central to quality improvement as we will see in Chapters 2 and 3, and must be given by any approach presenting itself as appropriate for health services. The answers are more difficult to find in public services than in a service where an individual walks in, cash in hand, asking for a service.

4 *The 'high intangibles' content of many health services.* Subtle behaviours of staff and the type of relationship which they establish affects the client's judgement of a health service, and often influences the 'cure' or efficacy of the treatment.

We readily sense whether other people are concerned about us and are interested in us. This sense is heightened if we are ill, vulnerable and dependent and need someone else's help. How staff treat a client in the general sense, indeed in many instances how they feel about the client, largely determines the extent of client satisfaction with many health services — it is the main thing which clients can and do judge.

The 'higher intangibles' content of health services, or 'relational quality' is significant when we wish to use some of the main methods of improving quality — specification, measurement and control. In manufacturing, quality is improved by physical specifications, by measurement of the product and by controlling variation. In services this is more difficult because there is often not a physical product to measure. Measurement is of customers' perceptions and of the cost of poor quality. In some services behaviours of front-line staff are specified and controlled (e.g. McDonalds, Disneyland), and attention is paid to measurement, specification and control of internal services.

It is possible to use these methods in health services but there are limits to the extent to which they can be used. This is because there is a greater personal service content of a particular kind. The link between staff behaviours, whether they care for the client and their feelings towards the client, are closer, or at least more apparent, to clients. Although behaviours can be specified, the source of those behaviours — the thing which clients sense — cannot be specified and controlled. Caring staff are an essential (but not sufficient) condition of health service quality, whereas this is not so necessary elsewhere.

Of course clients also value a professional approach, and many professionals argue that caring and feeling do not and should not influence how they treat clients. This takes us to the fifth difference.

5 *High professional component of health services.* There are areas of professional work where specification, measurement and control is commonplace and valued, but many areas where it is inappropriate and is strongly opposed. Professional discretion is necessary to decide treatment and in providing the service.

Closely related to this point is the fact that clients cannot judge the quality of significant aspects of the service. This is not just because they are often not in a fit state to do so, but because they are not technically competent to make a judgement. In fact many professionals argue that even their colleagues are not able to judge the quality of their work.

The willing cooperation of professionals is thus necessary, not only in relation to specification, measurement and control, but in order to judge one of the key dimensions of the quality of the service — to what extent the professionally-assessed needs of the client are met, and how well the service carries our professional assessments. Finally, the high professional component also refers to a large number of different professions, each with their own social systems and rites. Service quality depends on interprofessional cooperation, which is often hard to obtain.

Other differences are relevant but less significant for introducing quality approaches: local and national political control, changes to finance allocations, the number of central prescriptions, local community sensitivity, difficulties measuring outcome, and unevaluated or difficult to evaluate treatments.

If we are to realize the value of the quality approach in health services, these differences mean that we have to adapt established methods for improving quality or use them selectively and with care. The rest of the book describes ways of doing this.

Summary

Health services, and especially public health services cannot be viewed in the same way as most commercial services. In most commercial services an individual customer chooses the service from a wide range of alternatives, and explains what they want to staff. The income and future employment of these staff are directly related to whether they give customers what they want. The customer then receives a service from staff who follow specifications of what it takes to keep the customer happy. These staff did not have to be involved in formulating the specifications and do not come from different professions. The customer pays for the service and can easily judge whether they are satisfied with it and whether it was worth the money.

Health services differ in a number of respects. Quality approaches which offer frameworks and set strategies do not always recognize these differences. A common framework and strategy for quality is essential in even the smallest health services, but it must be one which is appropriate to the circumstances of that service.

Overview of 'Health Service Quality'

Chapter 2 discusses strategy and marketing. Getting these right is an essential precondition for using quality methods and techniques. It emphasizes the importance of a clear business mission and shows how to develop a service strategy.

Unlike many commercial services, public health services do not have to satisfy customer-purchasers, but rather purchasers, referrers, clients and often carers as well. Health services have to deal with more conflicts and more political and moral issues than many commercial services. This complexity means that the marketing techniques of segmentation and differentiation have to be used in certain ways to formulate a service strategy.

After this discussion of how to ensure that the right clients get to the service, *Chapter 3* then considers how to find out what they and their referrers think about it. It considers the first of three dimensions of health service quality: Client Quality. It explains why client, carer and referrer perceptions are important, and the different ways in which clients perceive services — in terms of what they want, what they expect, what they think they need, what they experience at different times, and their overall impression. The chapter proposes that a service should find out what is important to clients' choice of service and to their satisfaction once they receive it. It should then ask clients regularly to rate the service on those features which are known to be important to them. It describes ways to measure client dissatisfaction and satisfaction, the latter being more important in maturing markets. It describes a flow-process model for analysing the service from the client's point of view to decide where to make improvements.

Chapter 4 turns to the second of the three dimensions of service quality: Professional Quality. It discusses changes in client–practitioner relationships to improve quality and how to deal with conflicts between what a client wants, and what professionals think that a client needs. It examines methods for improving Professional Quality such as medical audit and peer review processes. It considers how to define Professional Quality standards for a service, and the issue of outcome standards.

Chapter 5 treats the efficiency of the service separately from Client and Professional Quality and as part of the Management Quality dimension. A service could give clients what they wanted and what professionals thought they needed, but it would be a poor quality service if it was wasteful and inefficient. Management Quality is about designing and operating the most productive and efficient service delivery processes. This chapter shows how improving Management Quality cuts costs and raises productivity, rather than lowering productivity, which is often the result of cost-cutting programmes. It also removes frustrations for staff, gives them control over their work processes and makes work more satisfying. The chapter introduces more quality methods for costing quality and problem-solving, and the Quality Correction Cycle. It considers the unquantifiable costs of poor quality, and shows how to calculate the return on investment of quality projects. Defining Management Quality standards completes the set of quality standards for a service.

Chapter 6 shows how to ensure that the service carries out and integrates improvements to the three dimensions of quality. It describes the Quality Management Cycle for continuous quality improvement and the methods to use in the standard-setting and measurement parts of the cycle. It shows how to use external requirements and internal analyses to set standards, and how to deal with conflicts between the three dimensions of quality. The chapter also shows how to choose methods for setting standards and measurement which are appropriate to the quality problems and the ability of staff to use them. It also explains more sophisticated methods for continuous quality improvement using statistical process control techniques.

There is a view that in the emerging health 'market' in the UK, health service standards would be protected and raised by accreditation. *Chapter 7* argues that accreditation through national performance standards does not assure quality for purchasers, does not encourage providers to continually improve quality, and does not contain costs. It explains more about the quality philosophy in a discussion of quality assurance and quality systems. It draws lessons for the UK from the experience of other countries that have used different types of accreditation.

Chapter 8 then turns to what is probably the most important subject for managers — how to introduce quality. It proposes that the tools and techniques for improving quality are as important as changes to attitudes, relationships and culture in the service. It argues for introducing quality in phases, and for developing a quality culture by linking in with staff concerns and motives and by using 'internal marketing'. It describes a 'top-down'/'bottom-up' quality strategy and outlines principles which give guidance for developing a quality strategy.

One of the themes of the book is the need to take a comprehensive and systematic approach to realizing the full value of the quality approach, whatever the size of the service unit. This involves using simple methods first within a Quality Correction Cycle and a Quality Management Cycle, as well as ensuring a balance between the Client, Professional and Management Quality dimensions. *Chapter 9* summarizes the book by describing a framework for developing a quality strategy and system — the 'Wel-Qual' approach. It concludes with three key considerations in introducing quality into a public health service.

The *Appendices* give a Glossary of Terms (Appendix 1) and a simple audit checklist for quickly assessing the quality of a service unit (Appendix 2). Appendix 3 explains a more sophisticated audit method which enables a management team to decide where to invest to improve quality, and to formulate quality strategy in a short time. This method (the 'Maps-Qual' process) can also be used to develop a common understanding about quality within a group, and a shared understanding of the problems which overcomes professional and departmental boundaries. Two versions are available: one based on BSI 5750 and one on the USA National Quality System.

Appendix 4 reproduces a survey questionnaire which can be used to improve internal services within larger units. Appendix 5 outlines a peer review process for involving staff in developing a quality system, setting standards and improving quality. Appendix 6 lists some key elements in the approaches to quality of three different quality specialists. Appendix 7 is a postscript giving my reflections as a researcher-patient just after finishing this book.

2

Business Strategy and Marketing

*T*HE CHAIRMAN REMINDED *the quality working group that they had three weeks left to finalize their proposal for a quality programme. There had been debate about where the programme should start. There seemed so much to do all at once, as the member of the group who had been finding out about Total Quality Management kept insisting.*

Someone suggested getting consultants in. Before the discussion got side-tracked into what happened to the last consultant's report, and how consultants did not understand the unique history of the service, the chairman asked some of the quieter members for their views.

One of the assistant programme directors said that, frankly, he was worried: all the discussions about what should be done seemed to assume considerable resources and time. Yes, quality would reduce costs in the long term, but working out the costs and expected returns of the different projects was missing the point. Staff already had to cope with a lot of other changes. More importantly, staff either did not believe in or did not understand why they were making all these changes. People were concerned about the future of the service and their own futures — there was talk that the reforms would mean more redundancies. They needed to be convinced that the quality programme would help get them and the service where it needed to be. And was that not the real issue — that we really did not have a clear idea of where we were going — a strategy?

Introduction

It may seem strange to start a book about quality by discussing business strategy and marketing. I do so because many quality programmes fail because an organization does not have a clear business strategy. The quality programme becomes a substitute for such a strategy. The programme does give staff a clearer purpose, but the service is not clear about its market and target client groups, and does not have clear business objectives and priorities.

Sometimes quality programmes are successful but produce high-quality services for the wrong customers — those not most in need, or the most profitable. In all cases a quality programme highlights any organizational inadequacies and lack of clarity about overall purpose. In the complex, newly-emerging health 'market' a business strategy is even more important to give staff direction and focus.

This chapter is not intended as a full discussion of business strategy or of marketing. These subjects are extensively and expertly covered elsewhere (Porter 1980; Kanter 1986; Peters 1986; Harvey-Jones 1988 for service organizations; Davidow & Uttal 1989; and for UK health services, Kinston 1988 and Shaeff 1991).

Those who have 'done' strategy and want to go straight to the discussion of quality may turn to the next chapter, which looks at the service from the point of view of the client when they 'reach the door'. What follows in this chapter is about deciding which clients should be guided to the service 'door', and the type of service they should receive if the organization is to compete successfully in a changing market.

The chapter starts by looking at business strategy in general and why health providers need one. It then concentrates on a key component of a business strategy, a service strategy. It looks at how one should be developed for a large NHS provider made up of a range of sub-services (e.g. a Directly Managed Unit (DMU), an NHS Hospital Trust (NHS-T) and some NHS trading agencies). The general principles also apply to a general medical practice with its range of sub-services or programmes, and to sub-unit services (e.g. orthopaedic services, or a department such as catering or physiotherapy within a unit).

The chapter argues that management must ensure the 'strategic quality' of each sub-service by formulating service strategy, before staff can work on improving operational quality. Management does this by defining the service's markets, target customers and the type of sub-services to be provided to compete successfully.

The chapter shows how to adapt and use commercial marketing concepts in the health 'market' to develop a service strategy — concepts such as 'segmentation', 'differentiation', and the service 'concept' or 'package'. These concepts help to identify the target client populations, define the set of sub-services, set priorities, secure contracts with purchasers, and attract the target clients by marketing to clients and to referrers.

Business strategy — general points

The success of a health service depends on all staff working to a common purpose and on a sound business plan. A business strategy statement describes the aims for the service, the plans for achieving the aims, and the values which support the means and the ends to be achieved. The core is a mission statement about why the service exists and what it is for.

> ### Business strategy
>
> A strategy provides a vision of the position the service wishes to occupy in the health marketplace in three to five years' time, and a statement of 'the business the service is in'.
>
> A business strategy defines:
> - The overall objectives and mission of the service
> - The different operational sub-services which are a necessary part of the service to achieve these objectives
> - Which support sub-services to be provided internally
> - The different client groups to be served by each operational sub-service, and priorities within these groups (segmentation)
> - What distinguishes each sub-service from others in what it offers to clients, referrers, purchasers and staff, (differentiation and competitive strategy)
> - The plan to realize the vision, including the finance, personnel, buildings and equipment plans and timetables (outlined in the Business Plan)

Some strategies fail because of a lack of understanding of the market, or over-optimism about ability to achieve objectives within cost. More frequently failure is because the strategy is known only to a few top managers or planners, or to a few partners in the practice and is not part of the life of the organization — it is only a statement.

As important as the technical quality of the strategy (e.g. phasing projects, cash flow projections, etc.) is whether a strategy unifies, orientates and motivates all staff towards a common purpose. A strategy must function as an organizing principle which gives sense and meaning to people's working lives. It must be congruent with values as well as giving guidance which helps people to make decisions.

Such 'living strategy', which is also technically sound, is created through staff involvement and a 'top-down, bottom-up' iterative cycle of discussion and debate — something which was missing with the tight timetables in the early stages of the NHS reforms. Strategy is made real by the process through which it is developed, by effective leadership, and by a culture which is consonant with the strategy.

In the absence of a strategy, a quality programme becomes the only thing which gives direction and purpose to the

The need for a business strategy

Without a strategy, and one which is clearly understood by all, it is difficult to decide how to invest to develop different sub-services, how to set priorities and workload, and how to present the service to the public and purchasers.

Without a strategy staff are not clear who are to be the priority clients and key purchasers, what they value, and what the service must do to meet their requirements.

It is also difficult to formulate a service concept or package which has meaning for staff and clients.

A simple process for developing and revising strategy is necessary because strategy is quickly out of date. It is also essential for obtaining staff commitment and the energy to make changes which will move the service in the direction it needs to go.

service — hence the temporary success of quality programmes in some services. However, it may be the wrong direction. In a changing market, simply doing the same things better is not enough.

Here we are not concerned with business strategy in general but with that part which defines who the service is for and what will be offered — the service strategy. This is because service quality depends on designing services for client groups with distinct needs — getting the strategic issues right. The focus below thus turns to service strategy, which is the link between general business strategy and operational quality.

Service strategy

A service strategy is based on a market analysis and a financial analysis of the services which can be provided to certain clients for the organization to remain financially viable and to prosper.

A strategy defines the type of services which the organization must deliver to compete successfully in its particular

Service strategy

That part of a business strategy which defines (a) the target clients of the service, (b) their needs, and (c) the type of services which are to be provided — the different 'service packages' or 'service concepts' for each target population or client group.

markets. Large organizations such as DMUs and NHS-Ts
are made up of different sub-services, each with different
markets.

Deciding which services to offer

The two key decisions in formulating a service strategy are
(a) which set of sub-services to offer and how to structure
them (i.e. grouping and design); (b) which sub-services to
expand and which to contract or discontinue. This chapter
considers the limits to the freedom which different health
providers have to make these decisions.

In the past these issues were influenced by a variety of
factors such as provider convenience, history and professional
preferences. The reforms brought a separation of purchasers
and providers, an emerging health market, and income following clients. In response, service providers have to make
explicit decisions and decide a strategy which is influenced
by referrer, purchaser and client views.

Three sets of ideas help a service to develop a more market-
orientated strategy. The first is the 'service success equation'
which shows the relationship between client needs and
service responses. The second and third are concepts from
marketing: 'segmentation' and 'differentiation'.

The next sections of the chapter present these ideas and
show how they help a health service provider to develop a
service strategy for the complex health market. In so doing
the discussion shows that quality is not just about giving a
good service, but is also about ensuring that those who need
it obtain the service, and ensuring that the overall design
meets their needs. Marketing and strategy in fact overlap
with operational quality issues.

The 'service success equation'

In commercial services there are two parts to the equation
which lead to profit (see box below).

1 *What customers want and the price they are prepared to
pay* for the service they want — the value to them of receiving
the benefits the wanted service provides. This partly depends
on what other services are already providing and their price
to the customer. A market analysis of customer demand and
existing providers gives the information to fill in the first
part of the equation, which is summarized by the term
'needs' in the equation in the box below.

2 *The service response or 'service package', and the cost to
the organization of providing it.* This part of the equation is

the type of service which could be offered to meet needs. An organization considers whether it can provide a service people will buy, and how much it would cost to provide this service. Putting the two parts of the equation together shows how much profit the service can make and whether to enter, expand or withdraw from the market.

The service success equation

Part 1: **NEEDS**   Part 2: **RESPONSE**
What customers   What service we can
want/Price they + provide/Cost to us = Profit or ·
will pay for it   to provide it   Loss

                    Relative to competition

We will shortly consider how this equation applies for a health service provider (e.g. directly managed acute or community unit (DMU), an NHS Hospital Trust (NHS-T), or a general medical practice). First we need to note some points about the two parts of the equation, and look at how commercial services decide which needs and types of customers to serve, using the concept of segmentation.

To illustrate the difference between needs and response consider an elderly person leaving hospital after an operation. They want help to get around the house, a supply of groceries, help with washing for the first few weeks, some company, help with financial affairs, and someone to call if they have a problem. They also need monitoring of their medication and general state. These wants and needs form the first part of the equation. The second part is the service response: a daily home help, meals on wheels (not what they wanted but the closest thing to it), and regular social work and district nurse visits.

This equation separates what people want (needs) from the service response to meet these wants (response). It is used below to discuss strategy in the more complex health market. But note at this point that needs are closely related to responses. The separation of needs and response is artificial: wants usually imply or are defined in terms of the means of satisfying them — there has never been a want without a means of satisfying it.

This point is relevant when we consider what customers want and the price they are prepared to pay for a service (most of the 'needs' part). This depends to a large part on choice and the services which are available in the market (the 'responses' available). When customers wish for a service which does not exist they usually think of it in terms of elements of existing services — in terms of responses, not in terms of their needs.

Providers often make the mistake of defining a need solely in terms of their means of satisfying it, for example a 'need' for a surgical service, or, 'the needs of this client are for a physiotherapist and a district nurse'. However, a necessary (but not sufficient) condition for innovation is to conceptualize needs in new ways.

Note also that in everyday usage the terms 'wants', 'needs,' and 'wishes' are used interchangeably. In health, what is termed 'needs' in the above model is made up of both what clients want and what professionals (including referrers) think that they need.

Returning now to our discussion of service strategy. Commercial services usually decide what services to offer by judging whether they can make a profit by providing a particular service to a defined customer population. To understand more about service strategy we now need to look at how commercial services decide which needs and which types of customer they will serve. More profit can be made by more selective targeting of customers and by packaging services to meet their specific needs. These ideas are embodied in the concepts of 'segmentation' (part of the first 'needs' part of the equation) and the 'service package' or 'service concept' (related to the second 'response' part of the equation).

Segmentation

The lesson from research into services is that, unlike manufacturers who can make a great variety of products (they do not just customize one product), few services are able effectively to provide more than one type or level of service. The secret is to decide which type of customers ('needs') to provide with a particular type of service ('response').

In health services this translates into defining different health needs and designing different types of service to meet these needs. It means defining the different sub-services to be provided by distinguishing distinct types of needs. In the past this strategic work was not done well. Where it was done it was driven more by provider convenience than client need.

In commercial services the essence of a service strategy is segmentation. This means identifying different types of customer so as to decide what service to provide for their specific needs (Heskett 1986; Davidow & Uttal 1989; Denton 1989).

Segmentation

'A service cannot be all things to all people ... Groups or segments of customers must be singled out for a particular service, the needs determined, and a service concept developed that provides a competitive advantage for the server in the eyes of those to be served ... Segmentation is the process of identifying groups of customers with enough characteristics in common to make possible the design and presentation of a product or service each group needs.' (Heskett 1986, pp. 8–9)

Davidow & Uttal (1989) cite the example of Shouldice Hospital near Toronto as an example of a successful strategy based on segmentation and design of the right service package for the targeted clients:

'By segmenting the market of sick people according to their complaint, then concentrating on a single segment, Shouldice has gained the ability to optimize its operations far more than general hospitals can. Its doctors have become highly proficient after doing hundreds of hernia repairs a year using Shouldice's special technique.' *Davidow & Uttal 1989, p. 49*

But be clear about why segmentation is so important in commercial services:

'But which customers are the best targets? Those who are the most valuable compared with the likely costs of serving them.' *Davidow & Uttal 1989, p. 38*

Segmentation in public health services

How relevant is the concept of segmentation to an NHS provider strategy? Surely a hospital or a community service has to ensure that its services are equally available to all? Can a public health service discriminate between clients in terms of which ones the service can make the most money from?

This is not the place to enter into the important debate about whether the UK health market will lead to worse services for 'unprofitable clients', as is already happening in some general medical practices (Sage & Kingman 1990). However, some discussion of these issues is important if we are to make the best use of research into commercial services, and of concepts such as segmentation.

There are two main issues. First, how free are providers

(DMUs and NHS-Ts) to specialize and to close services (related to the question of what is a 'core service'). Second, for a given range of needs and services, how can segmentation be used to decide how to group or structure sub-services and to decide the design of each sub-service.

In the first stage of the reforms, purchasers contract their own directly managed units (DMUs) to provide the same broad range of services as they did in the past. Contracts are based on client groups or specialisms, with providers making their own decisions about their support services. In this stage it is likely that DMUs will not specialize.

Segmentation is relevant here in helping to decide whether, or how to restructure a unit's sub-services. The range of sub-services offered and the nature and boundaries of each should correspond to different client/population groupings and their needs. Market research and segmentation analyses help to define these groupings and give a basis for a needs-based service structure.

The way contracts are sub-divided already points in this direction. Purchasers are dividing contracts more on the basis of client group/needs than on the basis of provider service structure. Segmentation methods offer a more systematic approach to defining client groups with distinct and homogeneous needs. Purchasers and providers can collaborate to undertake the market research and define segments rather than duplicating the work.

In the second stage of the reforms, purchasers will become more willing to contract providers other than their own DMUs, and more DMUs will become self-governing. The health market will become more complex, especially with GP purchasers, and prove intense provider competition. There will be more scope for providers to specialize, and more choice about which services they will provide. The situation becomes closer to the commercial example described above, although it is yet to be seen whether NHS-Ts will be allowed to reduce or close certain services.

In this second stage, market research and segmentation are important to providers' commercial success, especially as other providers will be using these techniques to decide different client needs groupings and to design and package services accordingly.

Segmentation in the UK health market

In the new UK health market, purchaser authorities are responsible for ensuring that equity and the needs of all the population are considered. The political and moral issues of how resources are allocated between competing needs and client groups are focused more sharply where they should be — with public purchasers rather than with providers.

The purchaser–provider split frees providers to concentrate on what they do well and for a low price and to develop their expertise. If the reforms work they will be rewarded rather than penalized for efficiency and for attracting more clients.

This ensures that in those markets where clients are able to and wish to travel they get a better service, which is also less expensive for purchasers. Where accessibility and proximity are more important, public purchasing authorities can influence local providers to provide a range of services, rather than to specialize in some markets.

However, purchasers may choose a provider more on the basis of cost than on, for example, proximity, if all other things are equal. The anomaly of public purchasers directly managing local providers with whom they contract does not necessarily mean that the purchaser will influence them to offer a range of services. They are just as likely to influence their providers to offer 'profitable' services.

Who is the customer?

The concept of segmentation can help to clarify the first part of the 'service success equation' if we recognize a further complexity of the health market. That is, who the 'customer' is and how needs are defined.

Unlike most commercial services, public health services do not have a simple customer who is a purchaser, who also knows what they want, and can judge whether they got what they wanted. In health there are a number of different definitions of need and different customers whose expectations have to be met.

In health services the first part of the service success equation ('needs' and the price customers are prepared to pay) is in fact made up from the following:

- What clients (direct beneficiaries) want and expect
- What carers want and expect
- What referrers (usually general medical practitioners) want for their clients
- What purchasers (who may be GPs) want

In addition:

- The price purchasers are prepared to pay for a service which provides all of the above.

The service success equation in health is as follows:

Needs		**Response**		
What is wanted by clients (and carers), and thought to be needed for clients by:	+	What service we can provide/ Cost to us to provide it	=	Survival or NHS-T surplus
• referrers				
• providers				
• purchasers/ Price purchasers will pay				

The key consideration is what influences a purchaser's decision to purchase, and hence the income to the service? The answer to this question is different for different services and for different purchasers.

Acute services

For most acute services, health authority purchasers are influenced by GPs' views, as indicated by referral patterns. The evidence is that what clients and carers want is less important, with some exceptions (e.g. maternity and oncology services). Where GPs are purchasers of acute services, GPs' decisions to purchase are likely to be influenced by their own views and the views of their patients.

The implications are that acute services whose income depends on health authority and GP purchasers should first find out GPs' views, and then those of clients and possibly carers. Research into GPs' views about different types of client needs is necessary to identify client segments. (In this book segmentation is used to identify client groupings, rather than referrer or purchaser groupings, whose requirements of a service are different.)

Non-acute services

For many non-acute services for elderly people and for children, health authority purchasers are likely to be influenced by carers' views, GPs' views and possibly clients' views. In the case of mental health services, purchasing health authorities are influenced by GPs, but also by other referrers, carers, clients, pressure groups, and by providers' perceptions of needs.

The situation is different for GPs (budget-holding or otherwise). The strategy issues for GPs are to attract clients to register with the practice, and to design a range of services which clients want and which the GPs' contractor thinks that clients need (the Family Health Service Authority (FHSA)).

In principle, market research is necessary to find out clients' preferences, identify segments and to design sub-services/programmes to provide what they want and to meet their needs. In practice most GPs cannot afford this research, and collaborate with their FHSA. The FHSA has data on needs and will identify client segments. This forms the basis for GPs to decide their sub-services/programmes, if these have not already been defined by specific contract requirements.

However, what clients want is also important. To make sure that they attract and retain clients, GP practices will have to supplement FHSA needs data with local market research before deciding their service designs. One study to assess needs in local communities using this type of approach is reported by Ong & Humphries (1990).

In summary:
• DMU/NHS-T providers need to find out the relative importance ('weighting') of these different views to purchasers' decisions to place contracts (ask them)
• DMU/NHS-T providers should do market research to find out what is important to GPs in their decision to refer, and to clients and carers in their choice of service
• GPs should collaborate with their FHSA (and DHA) to identify distinct needs in their area (needs segmentation), and do market research to identify different client groupings in terms of their different wants (wants segmentation).

Segmentation in formulating service strategy

Segmentation is 'the process of identifying groups of customers with enough characteristics in common to make possible the design and presentation of a product or service each group needs'.

For health service providers, market research and segmentation are necessary for three purposes:
1 To help to decide which sub-services to provide (or how to group specialties). The way sub-services are defined and structured should reflect client, referrer and purchaser preferences. Market research into how clients and referrers choose and use services helps to clarify

client segments. This information can be used to decide the type of services to be provided. Shaeff (1991) describes in detail different market research methods for this purpose.

2 Once each sub-service is defined with its target client segment, each sub-service should define the different types of client within the segment population. The sub-service must understand their various needs and design service processes specially for these different clients if it is to meet these needs effectively. The more a service can do this, the closer it can move to the ideal of individual and personal care.

For example, market research may discover that within a client group there are clients who have different needs for more or less information. Or the research may discover that there are clients with different 'participation needs' — some want to be active participants, others want to 'concentrate on resting' to get better. Further there may be evidence that outcome is improved by providing the right amount of information or participation. If this is known, services can be designed differently for those who wish to learn and participate. Segmentation on the basis of knowledge transmission and participation will become increasingly important.

3 The understanding of different needs which comes from market research and segmentation analysis helps to set priorities and regulate workload on a day-to-day basis. This is especially important at times of high demand and low capacity. Health services already segment clients in terms of urgency of need. In contrast to commercial services, once the type of client/need being served is decided, prioritization should be in terms of the client's needs, not in terms of how profitable the client is to the organization. Indeed, purchasers will want evidence that once the target population is decided, the service prioritizes by need rather than profitability.

So far we have seen how the concept of segmentation and market research methods help to decide which sub-services to provide, and give information for service design. The next concepts help to decide design, as well as which sub-services to develop. The concepts of 'differentiation' and the 'service package' relate to the second part of the service success equation concerned with the service response. After presenting these concepts the chapter outlines a set of steps for developing service strategy.

Differentiation, service package and competitive strategy

Differentiation is how the service 'stands out from the crowd'. Is differentiation needed in the health market? Is there a 'crowd' which a service needs to 'stand out' from?

In the emerging health market in the UK, two may be company, but three or over will be a crowd, and differentiation will be an essential part of a service strategy. It takes some time to differentiate successfully. If the UK health market does develop in the way intended, providers who have already established their distinctiveness will have a head start. That is, if the type of differentiation is right for the target segment.

Differentiation

Differentiation is how the service establishes in the minds of clients, purchasers and referrers what is distinctive about its response in terms of the benefits to them. A service positions itself in the market through differentiation. The aim is to achieve a competitive advantage.

Differentiation is entirely about how the important people in the marketplace perceive the service. We have already noted three sets of important people — clients, referrers and purchasers. The above discussion of segmentation singled out clients as the focus.

It is not sufficient to design and deliver services which meet target clients' needs. Clients have to be attracted to the service. Having identified a target client group, it is necesary to make an effort to differentiate the service in marketing to this group. In some health markets, clients' views may be critical to purchasers' and referrers' decisions (e.g. maternity and oncology services). In others, effort to differentiate the service in the minds of referrers and purchasers may be more important (e.g. surgery).

Just as segmentation can be made on any basis (e.g. sex, area of residence, diagnostic category, age), a service can also use any basis to distinguish itself from others. Examples are differentiation in terms of responsiveness (no, or short, waiting times), variety (e.g. many different specialist services in a DGH), superior professional quality, consistently high quality outcomes, or low price — but all only as perceived by clients, purchasers and referrers and in terms of the benefits to them.

The key to successful segmentation is to identify the 'best' clients for the service according to certain criteria. In the same way the key to successful differentiation is to choose the right way to distinguish the service in terms of what is important to the target clients, referrers and purchasers.

Many services make the mistake of trying to differentiate in terms of things which they think distinguish them from what they think are the alternatives, for example, by emphasizing their special techniques or equipment, or the training and background of staff, or the back-up facilities.

The service must have evidence about how important these things are to clients, purchasers and referrers before using them as a basis for differentiation. Usually if you ask clients about these things they say that they 'do not know the difference', in which case these are obviously the wrong bases for differentiation if their views are critical to referrers' and purchasers' decisions.

The source of differentiation never comes from the service itself. Differentiating criteria only come from the target clients, referrers or purchasers. The point is to find out how they distinguish services and to do so in terms that they use and that are important to them. Usually to create a perception of the service that is distinctive, the service must manage their experience of the service. This is difficult to do before they have used it. The most important thing is how the service initially presents itself and establishes its early relationship. We will consider these issues more fully in the next chapter.

One last point: a lesson from commercial services is that differentiation by price is a difficult strategy, and is rarely successful for long. The most risky strategy for a health service would be to distinguish itself from the competition primarily on price. It will be important for providers to understand how purchasers view the quality/quantity balance, and also to influence purchasers' views on this issue.

Differentiation by 'service package'

One way to differentiate a service is to develop the 'service package', either by developing a unique service package or by enhancing peripheral services. A service package is made up of a core service, which is the main service provided. The core service is the reason why the client is there (e.g. for surgery, or for an X-ray, or for therapy). In addition there are peripheral services which augment and enhance the core service (e.g. extra hotel services, the environment in which X-rays are taken, an information leaflet).

In mature and competitive markets there is frequently little difference between core services, and competition is in terms of peripherals (e.g. airlines). However breakthroughs are sometimes made by redefining the core service and developing a new service package or concept (e.g. a collection of alternative therapies in one centre). These breakthroughs are often helped by segmentation and by reconceptualizing client needs in different ways.

New service packages are one basis for differentiation through innovation. Another is innovation through new technology, such as CT scanner or laser surgery. However, differentiation by innovation is only relevant if the target markets value the benefits to them of the innovations — the tangible results.

A service strategy example

A community mental health team had problems meeting a growing and fluctuating demand and in deciding how to organize in the future. They did some research to find out the demands for the service, the different clients and their needs, the different sub-services they offered and their costs. This led to a decision to differentiate various sub-services in terms of three distinct client groups or segments — clients with acute psychiatric problems often needing emergency attention, clients with chronic and long-term problems, and neurotic clients.

Previously the team processed all clients through one system and tried to meet all needs by adapting one type of service. Their day hospital illustrated most clearly the failure of the approach. Disruptive acute clients disturbed other types of 'emergency' clients as well as the clients who were being rehabilitated into the community. Most clients with less severe problems simply refused to use the day hospital. The team developed a strategy which aimed to set a limit to the number of different types of client who could be served for a certain cost, and to develop specialist services for the three types of client.

They actively promoted the three services in terms of the benefits to clients, GPs and the purchaser of using the services. These were the benefits which they had found to be important to these interest groups, and which they guaranteed by setting limits to intake. (The health authority was able to use other services.) They also differentiated the service from others in terms of its specialist expertise for each of these groups, and by presenting the service as one which organized itself to meet individuals' needs, using the three sub-services to illustrate their approach.

Steps in developing a service strategy

The following draws together the concepts discussed above to show their part in developing service strategy. The box below shows where service strategy fits into the larger process of formulating a business strategy.

Formulating business strategy — steps in the process

1 **Service mission**
2 **Aims and objectives**
3 **Current services**
  Operational sub-services (each deliver one or more 'products')
  Internal support services
4 **Market and capability analysis for each sub-service**

Data gathering Assessing current and future demand, market shares
Current and future capability to respond, costs
Current and future competitors' performance

⎫
⎬ Service strategy
⎭

Analysis SWOT for each sub-service.

5 **Strategic decisions**
  • Understanding sub-service interdependence/synergy (e.g. could a sub-service be fully independent?)
  • Corporate issues
  • Combining analyses of each sub-service to decide which to expand/contract
6 **Change strategy**
  ('Turning the tanker' in the case of large units)
  and business and marketing plans
  Details, justification, and basis for control and reassessment.
7 **Implementation**
  Timetables, landmarks and responsibilities
8 **Review — return to mission**

This is not the place to discuss the details of business strategy, but we will consider practical steps for developing service strategy for a large unit because this is essential to service quality. The following shows how to use the concepts and ideas discussed above to develop a service strategy in steps 3, 4 and 5.

Step 3: current services

This step involves defining the different sub-services to be considered. The problem is that, in principle, a service should carry out market analyses first to decide which sub-services to offer and how to define them. But a service has to start somewhere, and most usually start by defining the sub-services which are currently provided, and by discussing with purchasers how they want services defined.

This can be difficult, because it is not always clear whether some sub-services are multidisciplinary or uniprofessional services. For many services, simply agreeing and defining each sub-service is an important step forward. The purpose of doing this is to be able to take each sub-service into step 4 and to carry out a market and capability analysis for each. (Step 5 then draws on these analyses to decide whether to redefine each sub-service, and which to develop and which to contract or close.)

Step 4: market and capability analysis for each sub-service

This step analyses the market for each sub-service (the 'needs' part of the 'service success' equation), and the capability of each sub-service (the 'response' part of the equation).

The market analysis involves market research to find out who wants and needs the sub-service and what is important in their decision to refer or use the service. Segmentation analysis helps to define client groupings with similar needs and wants, which is useful to redesigning the sub-service.

Market analysis also involves assessing current and future purchasing power. People may need and want a service, but there must also be a purchaser. Expanding into a market where there is need but no purchasing power is commercial suicide. It may be possible to use market research data on needs and wants to persuade purchasers to pay for more services or to buy new ones, but most purchasers' budgets are limited and they have to find finance from budgets for other services.

Thus the market analysis builds up a picture of amount, type and location of client needs, a picture of who might pay for needs to be met, and of the potential purchasing power of the market.

The capability of a sub-service is its current and future ability to respond to needs. This is assessed by gathering data about capacity, utilization, costs per client served, and costs of changing the service to better meet needs. Here decisions have to be made about service design (e.g. service concept or package) and which changes to make to compete in the market (e.g. differentiation). Often the constraint is not that purchasers cannot be found, or that purchasers would not be willing to pay a price which is necessary to cover the cost of investment to make the changes. Rather it is that investment finance cannot be secured.

As a result of this analysis the strengths and weaknesses of the sub-service can be assessed from the points of view of clients, referrers, purchasers and staff.

The final part of this step is to summarize these analyses for each sub-service by relating the capability of the sub-service to market attractiveness or potential. A 'business strategy grid' is used for this purpose (Shaeff 1991).

Step 5: strategic decisions

Even if the business analyses in step 4 shows that all sub-services have attractive markets and appropriate capability, the service has limited resources and cannot develop all sub-services at the same time. Step 5 brings together the business analyses for each sub-service to make the following decisions:
- Future definition of each sub-service (target clients, needs served and service design)
- Which sub-service to develop and which to maintain or reduce
- Which support services to contract out

This is the last step in formulating service strategy. The next steps of the business strategy are to decide the change plan, the marketing plan and the financial details.

End result of steps 3–5

The outcome of these steps is a service strategy with:
- A statement of the aims of the service in terms of the type of clients and their needs to be met in the future, and the type of sub-service which will be provided because it meets needs at the lowest comparative cost
- A statement of the distinctive features of each sub-service to be developed, which are known to be valued by clients, referrers and purchasers
- A general statement of each sub-service package, design of the service, and plan for developing it.

A business and service strategy sets the context for a

quality programme by defining the clients to be served. The quality programme can then focus on improving these clients' satisfaction with the service and on refining the service package — the subjects of the next chapters.

Summary

The emerging health market is neither as free nor as simple as many commercial markets, and never will be. It will take time for competition and choice to emerge and it is not yet clear how much specialization will be allowed. Although expectations are rising, clients, referrers and purchasers have no alternatives at present. The pressures to invest heavily in a service strategy are not as strong as for most commercial and freer markets.

However, providers without a strategy will be left trying to make up lost ground when competition does increase. Purchasers will, in time, have information about the needs of their populations and information about the responses offered by different providers. They already want to know how many of their population the service aims to provide for, and what it aims to provide at what price.

Providers must look at their costs, at needs, and decide what they are aiming to provide. They must consider what it takes to attract the type of client they aim to serve. Their income will be related to their success in attracting clients, and in particular clients whom they can serve effectively at a low cost in comparison to other providers.

Quality starts at the strategic level. Many complaints and waiting problems are because services attract and attempt to meet the needs of clients for whom the service is not designed. The range of needs is too varied, even for a service which is designed to be flexible. Success for most services in the health market will come from identifying distinct and homogeneous client needs (segmentation), targeting these clients to attract those most in need (promotion and differentiation), and designing services to meet their needs (service concept/package, and service process).

Once a service has ensured that it is getting the right clients (those whose needs the service is designed to meet at the lowest comparative cost) it may concentrate on operational quality issues — the subject of the next three chapters. Often quality problems in a service are due to poor strategic quality — not attracting and selecting the right clients and poor overall service design. There are limits to what staff at the operational level can do to solve these problems — they rarely have the time, skills and authority to address the strategic quality issues.

The successful services will not be those that provide

services which they think clients need. Rather they will be those providing what clients, purchasers and GPs say they want, and that use their information about needs to convince purchasers to place contracts. An understanding of these views is essential to formulating a service strategy.

A service strategy involves:
- Identifying client segments and their wants, needs and expectations
- Research into purchaser and referrer expectations
- Estimating what service can be provided, and costs
- Deciding which clients and services to concentrate on by building on service strengths to exceed expectations and cover costs. Identifying what will differentiate the service from the competition
- Developing a unique service package for competitive advantage
- Making sure that all staff, clients, purchasers and referrers are aware of what is distinctive about the service and its aims

*T*HIS CHAPTER LOOKS *at one of the three
dimensions of the quality of a health service, a
dimension which receives most attention in
discussions of quality and which I have termed
'Client Quality'. The chapter is concerned with what
the targeted clients of a service think about it, how to
avoid their being dissatisfied and how to increase
their satisfaction. It considers:*
- *Why service managers and staff should be
interested in what clients think about their service*
- *The cost of poor Client Quality*
- *How clients perceive health services*
- *How to set standards and measure this dimension
of service quality*
- *Practical steps for continually improving Client
Quality*

  *It shows how to consider a service as a process and
presents a model for analysing clients' experience of
the service and for identifying and removing the
causes of poor Client Quality (the 'Flow-Process
Framework').*

3
Client Quality

Introduction

The last chapter considered how a health service decided
which type of clients to serve, and how to ensure that only
these clients were attracted to and accepted by the service.
This is the strategic and marketing groundwork which is
a precondition for quality improvements by staff at the
operational level.

This chapter assumes that this work has been done and
that the service has got the right people to its 'door'. It
considers what those people and their referrers think about
the service, from when they 'enter the door' to leaving the
service and beyond. It introduces quality methods for changing the service to improve their satisfaction with it —
methods which ensure that cost-effective changes are made,
and continue to be made to keep the service ahead of
competitors.

The methods show ways of finding out which features of
the service are valued by clients, how to set Client Quality
standards, and how to measure clients' judgements of the
quality of the service. The chapter proposes that these
methods must be used by staff as part of a quality cycle to
ensure effective action and continuous improvement. It also
introduces the quality concept of the 'service process'.

Service quality means using these methods, but it also

means changes in attitudes and relationships. The chapter considers the benefits of a more equal relationship between clients and staff, where clients actively participate as 'co-producers' of a service, or 'prosumers', and where clients' expectations are frequently discussed and an implicit 'service contract' is 'negotiated' with each client.

Although the focus is on the general public as clients, most of this chapter is also relevant to internal services which have other departments or professionals inside a unit as clients. External Client Quality depends on the quality of internal support services. Support services must be clear who their internal clients are, what their clients want, and how to resolve conflicts between different client demands.

Who is the client?

In the last chapter we saw that success for commercial services in open markets lies in designing and delivering services which give customers what they want at the lowest price, and in persuading them that the service is better than competitors in these respects. Part of the quality approach is a set of methods for finding out what customers want.

Unlike most commercial services, health services do not have a simple customer-purchaser. To secure income in the particular type of markets in which they operate, large health service provider units have to satisfy the direct beneficiary (the client), carers, referrers (mostly GPs), and purchasers (mostly health authorities and budget-holding GPs). The income of the service depends on satisfying all of these people. Each service has to assess the relative importance of these different views to their income.

The situation is less complex for general medical practitioner services. Their income depends on attracting clients and retaining those registered with the practice, as well as satisfying their contractor-purchasers (the Family Health Service Authority). We also need to note that income depends on the decision to choose, and on the level of satisfaction with a received service. Some features of service which are important to a person's decision to choose are different from those which influence satisfaction once the service is chosen (see Fig. 3.1). For example, a long waiting time or list influences choice, but is less important or irrelevant to level of satisfaction with the received service. Note also that GPs' views largely determine choice (for large provider units), but once the client gets to the service, it is their views rather than the GP's that are important to future income.

The complexity of the health market means that large provider units such as DMUs and NHS-Ts have to take a two-stage approach. First attract clients to the service and

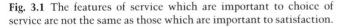

	Features critical to choice	Features critical to satisfaction
Referring GP	e.g. Waiting list Service unknown	Information Delivers on promises No unexpected after effects
Client	Distance Reputation	Hotel services General treatment by all staff Information understandable

Fig. 3.1 The features of service which are important to choice of service are not the same as those which are important to satisfaction.

secure income from purchasers. This involves (i) finding out what referrers (mostly GPs) and purchasers want; (ii) designing services to meet client needs, and (iii) pursuading referrers to refer and purchasers to purchase. The previous chapter covered these issues as part of service strategy.

The second stage is concerned with ensuring that those clients who do reach the service get what they want, and what they need. This is the realm of 'operational quality'. It is important because the future income of the service depends in part on what clients who receive the service think about it. If they are not satisfied next time they will go elsewhere or not use the service.

Thus the answer to 'who is the customer?' for a health provider is a complex one. The framework presented in this book considers quality to be more than just the end user's satisfaction with the service. It proposes that referrers mostly choose the service, and that purchaser contracts largely follow this choice. Their views are considered as part of the first stage concerned with service strategy — strategic quality involves attracting the right clients. Then operational quality focuses on those clients who do receive the service. It is concerned with whether the service gives clients what they want (this chapter) and with professional referrers' views about whether the service met the clients' needs (Professional Quality in the next chapter).

Client Quality

Whether the direct beneficiary of the service perceives the service as giving them what they want.

Carers' perceptions of the service are also important. The approach proposed here is to recognize that where carers are involved, there are two services being provided. In the example of services to elderly people one service is to the elderly person and another is to carers, even though the latter is often only an information or support service. These services may run in parallel for most of the time but they are distinct and should be recognized as such, and analysed as separate services. Each service will need to clarify the different services they provide to different beneficiaries, and the relative priority of each.

With these points in mind the rest of the chapter focuses on the direct beneficiary of the service (the client), recognizing that the same points apply to carers, who are a separate set of clients.

The costs of poor Client Quality

Why should people who work in health services be concerned about what clients think about their service? In the UK one declared intention of the 1990 NHS reforms is to widen choice and to make health services more responsive to clients. Although it is not a free market with a wide choice, one criterion purchasers use to decide where to place their contracts is clients' perceptions of providers' services. Health providers now have to consider the cost of poor Client Quality in a similar way to commercial services. It is therefore instructive to look at some of the research in this area.

The easily quantifiable cost of unhappy clients is only the tip of the iceberg. This cost is made up of the costs to the service of the time and money spent dealing with complaints, the costs of legal defence if the situation escalates, compensation payments in some cases (now exceeding 1% of some health authority budgets), and increasing costs of insurance. Providers are liable in negligence claims, and these claims are increasing. They have a financial interest in ensuring that clients do not advance claims.

However, the highest costs are the least visible to the service. Most dissatisfied clients are not moved to make a formal complaint, but simply try to avoid using the service again. One study of a range of services found that for each complaint there are about 26 dissatisfied clients, and this is in direct-payment commercial services where it is easy to complain (TARP 1980).

The study found that 65–90% of dissatisfied clients do not use the service again. Each dissatisfied client will tell between 12 and 25 other people of their bad experience (no doubt becoming more appalling at each telling). Each sympathetic listener will tend to choose another service if they can, or influence their referrer (e.g. GP) to do so if she/he can. Using these guidelines it is possible to estimate the custom which is lost to the service and which is difficult to get back, and to quantify this in terms of lost income.

The availability of alternatives is a key part of this costing equation.

Put this finding together with two other findings and the importance of avoiding dissatisfied clients becomes clear, even in public health services: a quick and effective response to a complaint ensures 95% return custom (TARP 1980). There is evidence that it also creates client loyalty that immunizes the client to the attractions of competing services. Secondly, it is far cheaper to retain existing clients than to attract new ones — strangely enough, advertising to existing clients is more cost-effective than advertising to attract new ones. Many companies now calculate and plan in terms of the lifetime value of a client — the value to the company of retaining that client and ensuring continued repurchases.

Readers do not need research but simply to reflect on their own experience to recognize some of these truths. How often do you go back to a service that was poor, especially if there is an alternative? In the last month, how many times have you made a mental note to avoid, or go to, a restaurant or hotel service which someone told you about?

Health providers need to judge how much their income depends on clients' satisfaction with their service. Is there a difference between health and other services in these respects? If there is, how long will these differences last? Health providers should also consider the effect in terms of costs of poor Client Quality on referrers' perceptions of the service. Although this chapter does not consider referrers' views as part of Client Quality, referrers are influenced by clients' views. One study found that clients' wishes in favour of a particular hospital/consultant were the second most important factor for 60% of the 24 GPs surveyed (Sargent 1991). The general points about the cost of poor quality also applies to referrers. Even one dissatisfied referrer may cost the service dear.

These costs are without looking at the income lost by not increasing satisfaction and the increased revenue accruing from high Client Quality. So far we have only considered the cost savings of avoiding dissatisfaction, but this is only one element of Client Quality. Increasing satisfaction is different — reducing complaints and avoiding dissatisfaction does not mean that clients are satisfied. It takes different things to produce satisfaction.

In competitive markets other services are continually raising quality. Actively seeking out what clients want and providing it becomes essential to survival. The cost of not trying to increase satisfaction continually is losing clients and ultimately going out of business. The reader must judge how far these points apply to health services, and to their particular sector.

The cost of poor client quality

- Poor Client Quality is expensive, far more expensive than some of the, usually minor, changes needed to avoid the most common causes of dissatisfaction
- However, reducing complaints does not necessarily increase satisfaction
- In competitive markets raising satisfaction is necessary to securing income
- The cost of not increasing satisfaction is lost clients (even if they were not dissatisfied), having to reduce prices, and lost income

Health providers need to understand more about how clients perceive health services in general and their service in particular, and make changes to respond to these perceptions.

Client perceptions of a health service

If we think about how we as clients perceive a service, for example a hotel or financial service, we recognize that our perceptions are formed in a number of ways. We only become aware of an aspect of service because we hold unconscious assumptions or conscious expectations which are, or are not, met when we experience the service. There are three types of assumptions or expectations.

Perception of a service in relation to assumptions or expectations

- Clients perceive a health service in relation to:

  1 *What a client wants from the service*, that is what they would like to receive from it, and what they feel it *should*, ideally provide. (Clients rarely ask for this from the service by making a *demand*)

  2 *What a client realistically expects the service will provide*, that is what they think it *would* provide

  3 *What the client thinks they need*, which may be different from what they want. ('I know its good for me, but what I really want is...')

- Often people are not aware of their assumptions or expectations until these are not met in their experience
- A client's *perceived experience* of the service will be different at different times (their satisfaction or dissatisfaction)
- This in turn will be different from their global and enduring perception or image of the service (their *perception of service quality*)

A client will have different assumptions about different aspects of a health service. For example they may perceive the type of medical treatment in relation to an ideal (the most advanced available and which they have read about), or waiting conditions in relation to 'realistic expectations'. These distinctions are relevant to deciding how to measure Client Quality and to understanding the importance of continually finding out and negotiating expectations. For example, when a client is asked to judge in-patient meals, are they judging against an ideal, or in relation to what they would expect from an NHS hospital, or what they think they need after surgery? It is important to be clear about what was measured because steps to improve Client Quality would be different in each case.

'No complaints' does not mean satisfaction

These points about client assumptions and expectations are most apparent with complaints. Complaints indicate clients whose perceived experience of the service at the time they complained was far less than what they expected of the service.

Although reducing the incidence of complaints is a good early objective for a quality programme (see Chapter 8), it would be misleading to rely on this indicator alone and incorrect to take it as a full measure of Client Quality. Clients may not be dissatisfied with a service, but this does not mean that they are satisfied. They may not be satisfied with it in comparison to what they want from it and feel it should provide — their comparison being another service or an ideal. Concentrating all efforts on reducing complaints will not raise Client Quality sufficiently in a maturing competitive market.

Even if most clients say that they are satisfied, they may still perceive its quality to be low, especially in public services. Frequently clients have low expectations and often do not judge the service in terms of what they want from it and feel it should ideally provide. Their experience of the service may well exceed their expectations, but they want more and feel the service should provide more. Knowing this is essential to the service to improve quality continually. Thus it is important to find out from clients what they would ideally like, and to seek out indicators of client satisfaction in ways described below.

Client Quality

- Is how clients perceive the service, which depends on their conscious expectations and unconscious assumptions
- Is influenced both by changing expectations and assumptions, and by making changes to the service
- A client is dissatisfied when their experience of the service is less than their expectations or assumptions
- Their expectations or assumptions may be in relation to an ideal, in relation to a similar service or to what they

think they are likely to get from a public health service, or to what they think they need

• Removing dissatisfaction will not necessarily increase satisfaction

• Client Quality is more than client satisfaction, which in turn is more than the absence of dissatisfaction

• A service must be clear about what it is measuring before deciding where to invest to improve Client Quality

Busy health service staff might find these distinctions over-subtle and playing with words, and certainly early on in a quality programme Client Quality should be viewed simply as client satisfaction. Strictly speaking, Client Quality is more than client satisfaction — it is a global and enduring attitude towards a service, built up from repeated satisfaction over time, rather than a judgement about the service in relation to a recent specific transaction. Again this is relevant in deciding what to find out from clients at a particular time, and in being clear what client feedback methods really capture. In competitive markets the focus turns from avoiding dissatisfaction to increasing satisfaction and then to influencing client-perceived service quality.

The practical implications are that service providers need to understand client's perceived experience of the service at different times, and to prevent incidents which clients do not like. Not only do providers need to improve clients' experience of the service, they need to manage clients' expectations to ensure that the service always meets or exceeds those expectations. The chapter shortly presents a method for doing this — the 'flow-process' model. First, we consider different methods for finding out client's perceptions, and how a service should use these methods.

Improving Client Quality

There is a variety of methods for finding out about and increasing clients' satisfaction with a service. However, if a service is to make significant improvements, the methods must be used as part of a systematic approach — as a part of a 'quality cycle'.

There are two types of quality cycle (Fig. 3.2). The first is the 'Quality Management Cycle'. Here, a service first selects the most important features of quality to define as standards, then measures performance against these standards, and then takes action if performance does not meet standards. The

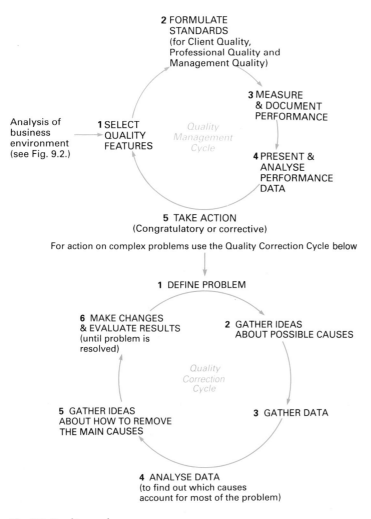

2 FORMULATE
STANDARDS
(for Client Quality,
Professional Quality and
Management Quality)

3 MEASURE
& DOCUMENT
PERFORMANCE

Analysis of
business
environment
(see Fig. 9.2.)

1 SELECT
QUALITY
FEATURES

*Quality
Management
Cycle*

4 PRESENT &
ANALYSE
PERFORMANCE
DATA

5 TAKE ACTION
(Congratulatory or corrective)

For action on complex problems use the Quality Correction Cycle below

1 DEFINE PROBLEM

6 MAKE CHANGES
& EVALUATE RESULTS
(until problem is
resolved)

2 GATHER IDEAS
ABOUT POSSIBLE CAUSES

*Quality
Correction
Cycle*

5 GATHER IDEAS
ABOUT HOW TO REMOVE
THE MAIN CAUSES

3 GATHER DATA

4 ANALYSE DATA
(to find out which causes
account for most of the problem)

Fig. 3.2 Quality cycles.

cycle is then repeated, with standards each time being revised
as quality is improved.

The second cycle is the 'Quality Correction Cycle'. This
is where a service picks a difficult quality problem and uses
quality methods to find out and remove the causes, and to
assess the results of the changes. The 'Quality Correction
Cycle' is often used in the later part of the Quality Management Cycle, to take action where quality performance is
less than the standard.

These cycles are explained in more detail in Chapter 6. They are introduced here before describing methods for finding out clients' views because a service can only make significant improvements to quality if such methods are used as part of a systematic process, not in isolation. The rest of the book develops this theme in different ways.

A good place for a service to start is to find out about complaints, and make changes by using the Quality Correction Cycle. Methods to measure client dissatisfaction are discussed in the next section. The section after shows how a service can take a more comprehensive approach by developing a set of Client Quality standards and starting the Quality Management Cycle.

Preventing poor Client Quality

Methods for measuring client dissatisfaction

The simplest and least expensive indicator of Client Quality is a regular count of the number of complaints over a period of time. Many services categorize complaints by type. Trends over time can be traced by keeping records and using a standard system to receive and document complaints.

One simple and effective method is for client-contact staff to have at hand a 'client dissatisfactions book'. They can be encouraged to note when they have not been able to provide the service the client wanted (which could be due to poor targeting and selection of clients to the service), or situations where they think clients have been less than happy with the service. This method has the advantage of involving staff in the improvement process and valuing their contribution, so long as improvements are made and staff are kept informed. The disadvantages are that it is an indirect measure and staff sometimes omit complaints which reflect badly on them.

These methods, like any others, are only any use if staff and management act on the information. This means using other quality methods within a correction cycle to remove the causes of the complaint (e.g. problem–cause analysis, Chapter 6). It also means that the culture must be one in which complaints or mistakes are welcomed as an opportunity to improve and to avoid the problem occurring for clients who do not take the trouble to complain.

There is a choice about whether to receive client complaints (and deal with them) outside the service, or whether service providers receive and deal with complaints, or whether both systems will be used. An external system may make it easier for some clients to complain, but it reduces the direct feedback from clients to the service providers. It makes it easier for service providers to deny responsibility — 'that's not our problem, you need customer services/patient relations'.

Service providers sometimes feel that if they give clients the opportunity to express dissatisfaction, then attention will be drawn to things they would otherwise ignore — that it is better to 'let sleeping dogs lie'. Generally the reverse is true: making it easy for clients to raise concerns at the earliest possible moment makes it less likely that they will make a formal complaint.

Research found that most complainants only wanted an apology and to be convinced that the same thing would not happen to other clients. One report is that 70% of incidents that progress to a lawsuit would not have done so if there was an early apology (Kent 1991). It is better to seek out possible dissatisfactions than let the situation escalate to anger or a formal complaint. This puts staff on the defensive, starts worries about legal liability if a mistake is admitted, and draws the battle lines.

More importantly, continually seeking out clients' views is part of the philosophy of negotiation and dialogue which is necessary to ensuring Client Quality. One way of judging how serious a service is about Client Quality is to look at the lengths the service goes to to make it easy for clients to give their views about it, and to let them know what action it has taken, for example by giving clients a list of standards and inviting them to judge the service against these standards (similar to 'our customer service pledge/promise'). Responses are higher if the service offers compensation to clients who can show that a standard was not met.

Increasing client satisfaction

Once a service has established ways of finding out about and remedying complaints, it may be more proactive and aim to increase continually client satisfaction. This means establishing a Quality Management Cycle.

Many services do not take this systematic approach. They start with an expensive survey to 'measure customer satisfaction' which gives a large amount of varied data. Although problems thrown up by the survey are discussed and changes are made, the effort is less productive than it could be, and is often not sustained. This is because (i) the responses to the survey mix features which are important to choosing the service with those that are important to satisfaction; (ii) the service does not find out which features of service are most important to most clients (relative 'weight'); (iii) the survey asks clients about things which providers think are important to clients; (iv) the service does not establish a Quality Correction Cycle or a Quality Management Cycle; (v) Client Quality standards are not set. The following describes a more systematic approach.

Step 1: Discover quality features

The first step is to find out quality features, their relative importance and 'threshold levels' for those who have received the service. People do not find it easy to define exactly which aspects of service are most important to them. They only become aware of these things when the service performs particularly well or particularly badly (see earlier section on perceptions of service). Consequently special market research methods are used to discover these quality features. These methods include:

• Focus groups. A representative group of clients is guided in discussions to find out valued features. (This method needs skilled group leaders.)

• Critical incident interviews and analysis. Asking people to reflect on their good and bad experiences of the service helps them to define particular features which are important. This technique is used in focus groups and can be used in semi-structured interviews.

• Flow-process analysis. Described at the end of this chapter. Clients are followed through the service process and asked about their experience at different times.

Step 2: Set Client Quality standards

The next step is to use this research to set standards. Chapter 6 discusses this in more detail. The basic principle is to take each feature of the service known to be important to clients, and decide how to measure it. The standard is defined as the level of performance to be achieved according to this measure.

For example, most services find that waiting time at the hospital for first consultations is a quality feature for clients. A measure of this feature is the time between the client arriving at hospital reception and seeing the doctor. A standard might be 45 minutes, set at this level because this met or exceeded most clients' expectations.

Step 3: Measure performance

The service then routinely measures performance in relation to the set of standards established. The most common method is a questionnaire which asks clients to rate the service on the features known to be important to them.

The most important step is the next part of the cycle — taking action to improve Client Quality. Chapters 5 and 6 discuss quality methods for deciding what action to take.

Measuring Client Quality

The last section presented methods for finding out what clients thought about a service as part of a Quality Management Cycle. The reason for presenting methods in this context is because many services set out in good faith to get feedback from clients, but this is not part of a systematic approach to quality and is less effective as a result. The point is not to measure quality but to improve it. It also distinguished between market research methods for identifying features of the service valued by clients, and their relative importance, and methods for getting clients routinely to rate the performance of the service on these features.

Many services find the market research too expensive. There are three other less expensive approaches. The first is to analyse the service process from the clients' point of view using the flow-process model described at the end of this chapter, and to pick out the quality problems revealed.

The second is to use research into clients' views carried out in similar services with similar types of clients, to decide which features to use for setting standards. The in-patient questionnaire developed by CASPE at the King's Fund College with Bloomsbury Health Authority is a good example of this approach in acute services (Kerruish *et al.* 1988). The King's Fund Quality Abstracts lists research of this kind in different services.

The third approach is to use research into a range of services to decide quality standards. An example is a USA study of clients of four types of service (see box below). The study found that clients all perceived the same ten different features of service to be important. A service could use this research to find out the relative importance of each feature.

Later research refined this list to the five features of Tangibles, Reliability, Responsiveness, Assurance and Empathy. From this the researchers produced a 22-item questionnaire which measures client expectations, their perceptions, and the gap between the two. The researchers propose that the questionnaire (SERVQUAL) gives a valid measure of client satisfaction in most services (Parasuraman *et al.* 1988).

Research into Client Quality features

The following features of service were found to be important to clients of four types of service in the USA (retail banking, stock brokerage, product repair and maintenance, and credit card (Parasuraman *et al.* 1985):
- *Reliability*
Keeping promises and consistency of performance
- *Responsiveness*
Willingness of contact workers to serve the client
- *Competence*
Employees have appropriate skills to perform the service
- *Access*
How easy it is to contact or get to the service
- *Courtesy*
Politeness, friendliness and client-orientation of staff
- *Communication*
Ways of keeping the client informed, in understandable terms, and interest in listening to the client's concerns
- *Credibility*
Trustworthiness, honesty and reputation of staff
- *Security*
Physical safety and confidentiality
- *Understanding*
Staff work hard at understanding the client's needs and concerns, and demonstrate their understanding in action
- *Physical tangibles*
Physical environment and appearance of staff and other clients

Other methods for getting feedback from clients

We have so far proposed that methods for finding out what clients think about a service should be used as part of a quality cycle, but quality also involves less formal and less systematic approaches — keeping close to and listening to the customer is a fundamental precept. The following lists other methods for getting feedback from clients, moving from the least systematic to more objective measures. Each has its use in different situations and each gives some indication of Client Quality.
- Talking to staff or clients about what clients like and dislike about the service
- Routine client-group or liaison meetings (used in some mental health, mental handicap, and family practitioner services)
- A letter sent to a sample of clients asking them to fill in

an enclosed sheet of paper entitled 'What I think about service X...'

- Mystery client (secret visit or use of service by assessor)
- Comments cards or questionnaire surveys
- Free telephone hot line for comments and complaints
- Observation against checklist (internal or external observer)
- Objective indicators of client satisfaction (e.g. demand, drop-out rate, client-cancelled appointments, a variety of service time intervals and waiting times, temperature, noise)

In summary, there is a variety of methods for finding out what clients think about a service. Each measures different things and is used for different purposes in different situations. The validity and accuracy of the method is not always the most important consideration. The choice of method should be influenced by its cost-effectiveness, its credibility and its likely use by service providers to make continual improvements and to judge the effect of their changes over time.

Any method of obtaining feedback is irrelevant if it is not used in a service which wants to find out and to make improvements. The culture and context must be one in which service providers are thirsty for feedback and want to act on the information. Given this, they will rapidly work out the best methods to use. The important thing is to use the methods as part of a Quality Management Cycle or within a Quality Correction Cycle.

Analysing the service process from the client's point of view

The discussion above introduced methods and concepts of the quality approach: measuring client perceptions and quality cycles. Two other principles of the quality approach are:

Service processes. Viewing the service and each person's job as a process — the series of activities carried out in succession to transform the client or material which is the subject of the service.

Customer–supplier chains throughout. Each worker or department has a customer and a supplier. Clarifying which internal (and external) services support the front-line service, and improving these services.

Understanding services in these terms cuts across professional demarcations and departmental boundaries, but is essential to improving quality. The following outlines a framework (a flow-process model) for analysing the service as a process. It is used here to show a cost-effective way for picking out areas of poor quality for the start of the Quality Correction Cycle, or for setting standards. It is also used in the next two chapters to analyse the Professional Quality and Management Quality dimensions of the service.

In manufacturing, the framework is used to construct the simplest and fastest production process and to trace delay and fail points (Øvretveit (EMI) 1988). It is used in the same way in health services. Here there are processes which transform objects (e.g. laundry) or information (e.g. finance). However, the object of most services is a client, who is usually a participant. Clients often co-produce the service, and they always actively experience the service and form perceptions of it.

Flow-process model

The flow-process model (Fig. 3.3) provides a framework for examining the service to understand clients' perceptions and to identify opportunities for error and fail points — points where problems frequently occur. The framework is adapted from a model by Johnson (1987). By tracing a typical client's career through the service from their point of view, it is possible to identify situations and encounters where the client may perceive the service to be poor. That is where their expectations are higher than their experiences. To improve Client Quality the service will need to eliminate problems which cause dissatisfaction, and take opportunities to manage clients' expectations so that the service can meet or exceed them.

The flow-process model is especially useful for helping staff to consider their service from the client's point of view,

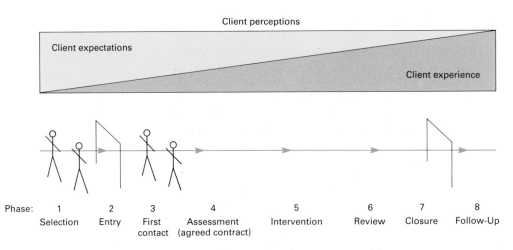

Fig. 3.3 Client Quality flow-process model.

and to gain a greater understanding of their part in the overall process. It breaks down the service into a series of steps which can be considered one by one. Service providers might like to try the exercise at the end of this chapter which uses this model to identify weaknesses in a service.

The process starts with the client and/or their referrer selecting the service — one of the subjects of the last chapter. The point of entry is where the client and/or referrer first contacts the service and makes a request.

Phase 1. Some client dissatisfaction can be traced back to the client or referrer selecting the wrong service. The service may attempt to help clients which it was not set up to serve well, or refuse to serve them and re-refer them after a long wait and without explanation. Publicity influences selection and expectations.

The quality of the selection process can be measured in terms of how many clients are turned away because they cannot be served, either because the service does not provide for their needs, or because it has insufficient capacity. Controls should include defining who is responsible for ensuring correct selection (e.g. marketing) and providing feedback about the type of clients who do contact the service — are they always the right type as identified in the service strategy?

Phase 2. The point of entry is where the client first contacts the service and makes a request (e.g. an entrance door or a telephone call). Quality measures include client perceptions of how easy it is to access the service and the usefulness of the information they were given at this point.

Phase 3. There is usually some delay and a queue between contact at the point of entry and what I have termed 'first contact', although entry and first contact may be the same thing. In some services reception selects the right staff or department to respond. This phase is critical because this is the first time the client meets a person representing the service. For a client who has a set of expectations, and who is anxious and uncertain about how they will be treated, this member of staff represents the service. They provide the client with the first real evidence about what the service is like, and what might happen to them.

This phase is an important opportunity to influence expectations and perceptions. For example, it does not reduce a client's anxiety or raise his/her confidence if staff do not know about a planned appointment, or expect the client at another time. Measures of initial (and subsequent) response times, of the conditions during the wait, and of client perceptions are important.

Phase 4. When a staff member receives the client and assesses their needs, the service makes its first substantive response. Poor assessment accounts for many quality problems. Much waste and dissatisfaction can be avoided by improving this phase (e.g. the right staff grades, training and assessment methods).

All phases are an opportunity for staff to find out what clients expect and negotiate what can be done, but this phase is the most important in this respect. Here the service provider, usually a professional, has the opportunity to encourage the client to talk in confidence about what they want and expect from the service. Service providers can bring the client's expectations into line with what the service can offer, which is critical to avoiding dissatisfaction. This involves establishing a particular type of relationship with the client. Assessment should in fact be a dialogue between service provider and client, involving negotiation and an implicit, sometimes an explicit, contract.

Measures are of client perceptions of the response, of staff skills and abilities to handle the needs presented, and whether the response is adequate to enable the next part of the process to be carried out: the intervention phase. Again there may be unnecessary and unwanted delays between assessment and intervention phases.

Phase 5. The intervention phase is where the service attempts to meet the client's assessed needs. It involves many points of personal contact which are critical for shaping the client's perceptions. Measures include the service's ability to meet adequately the different needs of the clients who have reached the intervention phase, and the time intervention takes.

Phase 6. The review phase is important for three reasons. First to reassess needs and replan interventions to have the maximum effect. Second to check client expectations and influence these, and third for service providers to judge whether their skills could be used to a better effect for other clients awaiting the service.

The client may want and expect continued intervention, but the service may judge that the client's needs have been met. Service providers may judge that other clients would benefit more: reviews provide an important link back to second-order Client Quality. That is, to ensuring that the service is available to all those who could benefit from it. Reviews are not purely clinical — they always involve opportunity–cost considerations.

Phase 7. The closure phase should be considered in terms of how clients experience this part of the service and whether they are properly prepared in all respects to leave the service. The service should check whether the client's wants and needs have been met (judge and record Professional Quality), and what action to take if they have not.

Measures of the quality of this phase include numbers of clients who left before this phase, as well as clients' perceptions of how their departure was handled. Sometimes closure also involves handover, for example to a community nurse. Just as delays and poor perceptions can be caused by poor internal services to the front-line process, so too can dissatisfaction be caused by poor handover to external services. A good general perception of a service can be destroyed by an external service not taking up their responsibilities.

Phase 8. Finally a follow-up phase involves the service checking whether the client's needs were met, and, if appropriate, pursuing opportunities for return or wider custom. This can involve calling referrers and documenting and acting on their comments about the service.

The above model is deliberately oversimplified in order to present a framework for analysing a service from a typical client's point of view, and to introduce the principle of viewing the service as a process. It suggests that delivery is a simple one-system process, which is rare. Service providers using this framework to analyse their own service will find that delivery involves a number of internal services and separate processes (e.g. admission, X-ray, ward stay, treatment, attendance at outpatient clinic). Many of these may involve the client, with a point of entry, assessment, intervention, and departure. Most quality problems occur between these processes rather than within them.

The processes may operate for the client in succession, with the client passing through one to another (e.g. diagnostic and therapy services at a DGH). There may be alternative services available at the point of entry and operating in parallel. (The Client Quality of internal services can be measured using the internal service quality survey reproduced in Appendix 4.)

The model helps service providers to clarify the boundaries of the different service processes, to clarify which services they are responsible for, and whether clients' expectations of what they are about to receive are formed correctly by other services. More sophisticated methods for tracing client flows and decision-making are useful for designing or re-designing services (Shostack 1984). This is often necessary when an initial representation using the above framework reveals a far-too-complex process which is trying to serve too many different types of client.

The flow-process model — summary

In summary, one of the central concepts of the quality approach is to view a service and each person's work as a process. The above framework can be used with staff in any service to:

• Help staff understand how the service works and their part in it
• Work out simpler and faster ways of bringing together clients, information, materials and staff (e.g. removing 'bottlenecks')
• Establish procedures for what should be done
• Raise staff awareness about how clients perceive the service
• Understand how staff can elicit and negotiate expectations to ensure that clients are never dissatisfied, and are, ideally, satisfied with the service

Following a few real clients through the process and recording their experiences is a more cost-effective method than questionnaire surveys, and gives information which clearly indicates problem areas in the service.

Finally, using this model produces a list of problem areas which can be used to define quality features and set standards for the Quality Management Cycle (Chapter 6), or for the start of a Quality Correction Cycle (Chapter 5).

Practical steps — how to raise the Client Quality of a service

It is easy to find out the main causes of dissatisfaction and to remove many without much expense. The steps to be taken depend on the stage of quality evolution reached by the service (see Chapter 8). The following is a summary of the main steps:

• Start by removing the main causes of dissatisfaction, and establish the Quality Correction Cycle as the systematic way to remove quality problems once and for all
• Involve staff in analysing the service as a process
• Get staff to ask clients what they expect and to negotiate what can be provided at every phase of the service process
• Use the process analysis to identify where the service goes wrong from the client's point of view, to set standards, and to select problems for the Quality Correction Cycle
• Use market research methods to find out what is important to clients — the Client Quality features
• Set Client Quality standards for these features
• Frequently ask clients to rate the service on these features — formally through questionnaires or informally in everyday contact with them

- Take action where clients rate the service as poor, using the Quality Correction Cycle

Service quality, however, will not be improved just by focusing on Client Quality. What clients want may not be what they need, and clients may not be aware of process problems which drain resources. It is to these other aspects of quality which we now turn in considering the Professional and Management Quality of a service.

Summary

People are beginning to judge health services by comparing them with the improved services they have come to expect in other sectors. If a health service responds to client wants and expectations it attracts more clients, and in many cases more income. Client satisfaction is important to purchasers' and referrers' decisions about contracts and about where to refer.

The cost of dissatisfied clients is high. For each dissatisfied client who complains there are many who do not, but who tell other people. This is the worst publicity the service can get, leading to lost clients and income as alternatives become available — a loss of which the service is rarely aware.

Avoiding dissatisfaction does not ensure satisfaction, although it is a good place to start. For example a clean and comfortable environment helps to avoid dissatisfaction and comes to be expected, but it does not create satisfaction. In a competitive and maturing market the aim is to find out what would increase satisfaction, and make continual improvements to stay ahead of rising expectations.

The pressure to increase client satisfaction in health services is less than in other services, in part because people's expectations are low in comparison with what they would like from the service, and they are reluctant to complain. Methods for obtaining feedback should be suited to the clientele. The aim is not just to get feedback, but to get the kind of feedback which is of most use to the stage of quality evolution the service has reached.

Using any method naturally raises expectations. It is also a waste of money if the service does not act on the findings. The context in which the method is used — one in which staff are concerned to make improvements — is as important as the method. The methods should also be used as part of a Quality Correction Cycle or a Quality Management Cycle.

It is better to use a variety of methods to measure Client Quality than to rely on one method, but even better to select the most cost-effective methods. This involves understanding what each method measures, the advantages and disadvantages of each, and the likely enthusiasm of staff for collecting and using the information.

Exercise: improving Client Quality

Purposes of the exercise:

● *To introduce staff to thinking of the service as a process, and from the client's point of view*
● *To identify situations where clients may perceive the service to be poor (Client Quality problems), and where there are opportunities to bring expectations in line with what the service can provide*
● *To serve as a basis for specification of the service (see Chapter 7).*

1 Using the flow-process framework, list on a flip-chart the main phases a typical client passes through in their contact with the service.
2 Represent the service delivery process using a diagram similar to the framework and listing each phase. (If this cannot be done, or starts to get too complex, it may be that the service delivery system is poorly designed or that client selection is poor — one process trying to serve too many different types of client).
3 For each phase, list things that go wrong, or are likely to go wrong, which may cause clients to think badly of the service. Where does the service fall short of reasonable expectations? (Client Quality problems).
4 Which of these problems causes the greatest dissatisfaction for most clients? Rank order the problems giving a '1' for the problem which, if eliminated, would do the most to improve clients' perception of the service.
5 Consider the causes of each problem and the cost of solutions.

---

*O*VER HALF OF *the 646 consultant orthopaedic surgeons who replied to a survey in the UK in 1989 said that they had been, or were being, sued for negligence. Over a quarter already had cases settled against them (185). 8% of these cases were 'wrong side/digit operation', 10% 'missed fractures', and in 18% of the cases the problem lay in the nature of the surgical technique. Although most of the causes were not said to be due to inadequate skill or knowledge on the part of the consultant or their junior doctors, 8% of the causes were due to wrong conclusion on examination, and 9% were due to inexperience or ignorance of a particular condition. The only responses to the 236 cases was minor expenditure on surgical equipment and three extra doctors.* (Survey reported in Health Services Journal, 29 March 1990)

With Health Authorities and providers meeting the cost of claims largely out of annual revenue, the future predictable cost of poor quality amounts to the closure of a number of wards or small hospitals in each district in the UK every year. One estimate is that the likely cost of negligence claims already being pursued will account for 13% of total health expenditure in 1996.

4

Professional Quality

Introduction

This chapter considers Professional Quality, the second of the three dimensions of the quality of a health service. Why do we need to consider Professional Quality as a separate dimension?

Clients are not the only judges of the quality of a health service

A health service could give clients everything they want, and could do so at a low cost and without waste. Would we then say that the quality of the service was high? In fact such a service might not properly assess clients' needs, and might not diagnose underlying illnesses.

The service might give popular but ineffective or even harmful treatments, or it might give the right treatment in the wrong way. It might carry out unethical procedures or practices, and might do many other things of which patients or managers were not aware, but which most professional practitioners could show were ineffective, unethical, or not in clients' long-term interests.

Although practitioners only advise patients about which treatment to undergo, clients are not the only judge of whether a health service would or did meet their needs. Even though the client and the professional should both be involved in deciding the treatment, it takes a professional to judge whether the best treatment was used, whether it was carried out correctly and ethically, and whether professionally assessed needs were met. In this respect health services differ from commercial services. This is one reason to assess the Professional Quality dimension of the service separately. Another reason is that special approaches are needed to improve Professional Quality (e.g. professional audit) which are directed and carried out by professionals. The best way to introduce quality methods is to help professionals to take responsibility for improving the Professional Quality of the service.

Professionals are experts in the procedures and in the details of what needs to be done. They need to be able to make the improvements which they know are necessary, and need help and encouragement to use new, more systematic and effective methods to identify and resolve priority problems.

Professional Quality defined

There are two related components to the Professional Quality of a service.

Professional Quality

Outcome: (1) Whether the service meets the professionally assessed needs of its clients, and
Process: (2) Whether the service correctly selects and carries out the techniques and procedures which professionals believe meet the needs of clients

The first component is judged by assessing outcome. There are many ways to measure the effects of a health service on clients. They range from a battery of measures in an evaluation study, to one or more professionals' judgments of the effects of the service. (The client's and carer's judgements of outcome are at least as important, but they are not included in this dimension of the quality of the service.)

The simplest measure is a rating by both professional provider and professional referrer (e.g. a GP and a surgeon or therapist) of the change in the client's presenting condition that can be ascribed to the intervention made by the service.

More sophisticated techniques are being developed for routine assessment of outcome, as well as performance indicator data bases. How a service could develop outcome measures is considered below.

The second, 'process,' aspect of the definition is concerned with how well professionals carry out assessments, treatments and other procedures, and with the effectiveness of these interventions.

'Techniques and procedures which professionals *believe* meet the needs of clients', refers to the fact that many health service treatments are based on clinical experience and tradition — many have not been scientifically evaluated. One of the biggest quality costs in health services is due to continuing use of discredited or outdated treatments.

This part of the definition recognizes that there is no point in carefully following procedures and setting standards for interventions which are of unproven benefit. It recognizes that health service quality would be significantly improved by a more rigorous evaluation of techniques and by developing treatments on a more scientific basis.

We may not have sophisticated routine outcome measures or evaluated treatments for some time. Hence this second part of the definition recognizes that the best thing we can do to ensure the right outcomes is to apply properly the assessment techniques and treatments which are believed to be the most effective.

Most services can do little to change 'believed by' to 'proven' because they cannot afford scientific evaluations. But they can ensure that professionals are up to date with recent research and regularly review and change the methods they use in the light of research. Where there are techniques and treatments which are proven and effective, then Professional Quality depends on how well professional providers select and use them.

Improving Professional Quality

The Professional Quality of a service is improved by enabling professionals to carry out professional audit, and by general managers helping to make changes arising from the audit. There are many types of audit, even within one profession, but all have in common a systematic approach to identifying quality problems, and to making and evaluating changes. Before considering types of audit, some general introductory points need to be made.

Assuring Professional Quality

Assuring Professional Quality means ensuring that staff are knowledgeable and skilled in the range of techniques necessary to assess and treat the type of client served. It means ensuring that they use these techniques properly, that there are professional procedures and policies, and that there is supervision or colleague support to give guidance. This aspect of Professional Quality is usually assessed and improved by professional audit.

In principle, Professional Quality is improved in the same way as Client Quality: in a systematic way using methods in a quality cycle. Some audit approaches choose a subject and use a version of the Quality Correction Cycle to gather data, analyse causes and evaluate changes. There are different methods for selecting a subject for the correction cycle.

Other audit approaches are more comprehensive and establish a range of professional standards, measure performance on each and take action where performance is poor. This approach is a Quality Management Cycle focusing on the Professional Quality dimension of a service.

From the point of view of service quality there are two drawbacks to most audit approaches. Whilst audit is systematic it is partial. The focus of medical audit is medical practice (DoH 1989) defined as, 'the systematic, critical analysis of the quality of medical care...', or 'the attempt to improve the quality of medical care...' (Marinker 1990). The most serious quality problems are often between professions and departments (e.g. communication and coordination) but audit is usually uniprofessional and is poor at tackling cross-profession problems.

Multidisciplinary team audit is being developed, but team audit approaches share another limitation. This is that audit rarely considers Client Quality or Management Quality. Although other staff can examine these dimensions of service, effective quality assurance brings the three dimensions together in a comprehensive quality system (Fig. 4.1).

The culture and organization of health services is such that there are good reasons to encourage each profession to develop their own audit arrangements in the early stages of a quality programme. However, at some point the service will have to consider how to relate these audit activities to other activities for improving the Client and Management Quality dimensions, and whether to run different professions'

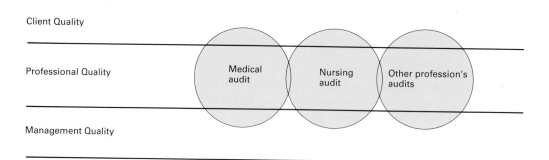

Fig. 4.1 The scope of professional audit. (Professional audit does not cover all aspects of the quality of a service.)

It is here that approaches to audit impinge on the question of unit management structures and the role of general managers. Service quality presupposes a team approach and common objectives. The way in which quality has been translated in health services reflects the complex and often unclear professional structures, and the power of professions. It is possible that organizational changes towards medical directorates and community teams may make possible comprehensive multidisciplinary audit, but uniprofessional audit may still be necessary in some services.

Uniprofessional or team audit?

The Professional Quality of the service depends on professional practitioners and departments reviewing and improving their practice using quality methods. It also depends on professions collaborating to overcome interprofessional quality problems such as poor communications.

Reasons for uniprofessional audit

Although many quality problems arise between departments and services, there are good reasons for each profession developing their own audit arrangements in the early stages of a quality programme:
- Audit is unfamiliar and threatening to many practitioners
- Audit should be part of the ordinary management process, and many services are structured primarily by profession
- Most experience with audit and proof of the value of audit is within each profession.

This experience, and colleagues' successes, help to get practitioners interested

---

Reasons for starting with separate single-profession audit include:

1 *Systematic and effective audit is unfamiliar and threatening* to many practitioners and often difficult to introduce. Even within a single professional group there are differences in views about the criteria of good practice and outcome, and a feeling that others do not properly understand or value an individual's approaches. I have found it even more difficult to introduce audit in multidisciplinary groups, where these differences in view are compounded by different pro-

fessional cultures, suspicions and jealousies (Øvretveit 1986). It is better to start by allowing practitioners to become familiar with audit approaches and build up confidence within their own professional group.

2 *Audit should form part of the management structure and process.* Education or supplying information alone rarely changes behaviour, even in the few cases where poor performance is due to lack of knowledge (Asbaugh & McKean 1976). To ensure that the improvement actions agreed as a result of audit are implemented, audit should be part of the ordinary management process. Many services are currently structured by profession: In fact the primary function of the professional structures retained in one service restructuring was to introduce and develop professional audit (Øvretveit 1990).

3 *Most experience with audit is within each profession.* This experience helps to get practitioners interested and to develop their own approach. Generic quality systems are rarely taken up by professionals. For example, Wilson (1987) reports problems involving doctors in a single hospital-wide quality programme in North America — problems due to fierce independence, poor participation and confidentiality.

Each professional group's audit arrangement should have ways of noting and addressing quality problems which involve other professions. That is, either problems caused for them by other professions, or problems which other professions bring to them. Inter-professional issues should be addressed by liaison members within audit groups, and by establishing Inter-Professional Quality Groups, whose function can develop in later stages to establishing multi-disciplinary audit.

With these points in mind, and recognizing the limitations of professional audit, we can turn to looking at what we mean by audit, the different types of audit and how to go about introducing audit. The discussion concentrates on medical audit because other profession's audit methodologies follow similar principles and because audit of medical practice has been the most closely studied.

Medical audit

In most services doctors already review practice in post-graduate lectures, case presentation, ward rounds, and in complications, morbidity and mortality meetings. Most of these, usually informal, activities concentrate on individual cases. They do not use systematic techniques to ensure that service improvements are made and evaluated.

In contrast, formal audit uses systematic or scientific methods to establish explicit criteria for good practice, measure performance, select cases, compare results amongst peers, and to decide and implement improvements. It also involves recording the audit procedure and the results of audit.

> **Medical audit**
>
> A systematic process for improving clinical outcome by (i) comparing what is done with agreed best practice, and (ii) identifying and resolving problems in the service delivery process.
>   Audit is the same as any approach to improving quality — a systematic and scientific approach with documentation, specification and measurement and evaluation of improvement actions.

Sophisticated approaches to audit involve professionals agreeing what constitutes the best practice in terms of outcome criteria and indicators, and in terms of how to carry out assessments and treatments (process criteria). Professionals select cases from their work and compare them to best practice. They investigate why there are variations from best practice and what improvements to make. Audit then involves follow-up and evaluation to find out whether improvements were made and whether they were effective. Through this approach, professionals increase their understanding of their service delivery process, of where problems occur, and where they need to make particular efforts to avoid problems.

Seven-step audit

One approach which gives an idea of what is involved in audit and which embodies the key principles is that reported by Dixon (1989). Dixon proposes that the approach allows for the cost-effective review of large numbers of cases in a statistically reliable way, without a computer and without needing large amounts of doctors' time. Dixon describes seven steps (which correspond to the Quality Correction Cycle model):

1 Design: select audit subject, specify objectives, and select patient group

2 Decide indicators: decide how patient care is to be measured in relation to audit objectives and data collection methods

3 Collect and organize data: audit assistant screens cases against indicators

4 Analyse data: cases not conforming to audit indicators are identified and analysed by doctors
5 Identify problems and causes
6 Take action
7 Follow up to find out if the problems were overcome

Examples of medical audit

The following examples and studies of medical audit show some of the benefits and outcomes, and can be used to encourage doctors to establish their own system.

Sellu (1986) reported simple but effective steps taken at the weekly surgical meetings of the general surgical unit at Ealing by presenting comparisons of mortality and morbidity data. Once variations in wound infection, pressure sores and length of stay were recognized, action was taken to agree criteria and improvements were made. Infection rates were reduced by 50% over 3 years, with estimated savings of £23 000 per year.

Young (1980), and Fowkes *et al.* (1986) report examples of audit which improved Management Quality by reducing costs, as well as improving Professional Quality. Studies of the use of tests and investigations in these audits led to improved assessment procedures, with fewer tests and better patient care.

A well known and successful example in the UK is the Lothian surgical audit, involving over 30 consultants. The audit resulted in reduced re-operation rates and less extreme surgery, and reduced operative mortality for large bowel resection for benign disease, biliary and pancreatic surgery and aortic aneurysms. Better outcomes were achieved in specialist units, especially for prostatectomy, vascular and breast surgery — the audit led to more cross-referrals between specialist surgeons (Gruer *et al.* 1986).

Types of medical audit

Medical audit methods can be classified into four types, each following one or more of the principles described above and each with their advantages and disadvantages.

Internal retrospective audit is the simplest and most common in the UK. The audit is internal to a specialty or hospital and uses past patient records and other records. One example is a retrospective audit of 100 patients admitted to a neurosurgical unit (Sandeman & Cummins 1986). It established that 96% of cases of extradural haematoma could be identified by junior staff with improved procedures.

External retrospective audit is undertaken by, or in cooperation with, one or more outside groups. The best-known example is the Confidential Enquiry into Maternal Deaths, which produces a 3-yearly report analysing causes of avoidable deaths (DoH 1989). The Confidential Enquiry into Perioperative Deaths carries out a similar review of deaths caused by surgery (Buck *et al.* 1987, and NCEPOD 1989).

Concurrent active audit is a review of the care of patients still under care. Such reviews are usually conducted in relation to established procedure or protocols for patients, or in relation to clinical plans. This type of audit is common in the USA, for example in utilization review, and where the necessary computerized information systems are established.

Criterion-based audit involves agreeing explicit and measurable criteria of good practice for selecting cases, and for comparing what is done against these criteria. Usually the criteria are only for screening records to select cases that do not meet the criteria for more detailed investigation. In countries using this approach other than the USA, criteria are agreed and applied in a number of hospitals, thus making it possible to compare performance.

Audit in general practice

All general practitioners are expected to be involved in audit by 1992, supported by a medical advisory group in each FHSA, which also involves hospital doctors (DoH 1989). Audit in general practice frequently engages issues of practice organization, but the focus is medical care of individual cases, or of a particular patient group. If competition increases there will be incentives for general practices to extend audit to cover Client and Management Quality dimensions, and to develop a comprehensive quality system as outlined in Chapter 6. Multidisciplinary audit will be necessary for some subjects (e.g. patients with mental illness, elderly patients).

The choice of audit subject is important because a general practice has limited resources and time, and it is never possible to audit all conditions. A simple start is to gather data to check that the practice is meeting contract requirements. Then the practice can go on to examine how they handle certain conditions. Here the aim is to maximize the chances that chosen 'tracer conditions' to audit will demonstrate how the practice deals with other conditions, and will highlight more general issues.

Dury and Styles (in Marinker 1990) suggest that chronic conditions including hypertension, epilepsy, asthma and diabetes mellitus are likely to meet the following criteria for choosing a tracer condition: high prevalence rate, easy to diagnose and well defined, suitable treatment has demonstrable effect, and non-medical factors in the condition are understood.

An example is audit of diabetes, reported by Kemple and Hayter (1991). This involved a retrospective audit of all diabetic patients in one year (223 out of 13 200) by examining their records against agreed standards (e.g. serum fructosamine and blood glucose levels, review according to protocol, and education of new patients). A medical assistant spent 110 hours on the audit (the authors do not report their time and practice meeting time), which found that many standards were not met. Changes were subsequently made to protocols.

Data collection for many audits can be delegated to practice staff. Essex and Bate (1991) found that a receptionist could audit immunization numbers, action in response to abnormal cervical smears, hypertension and smoking records, diabetic follow-up, reviews of serious mental illness, numbers of elderly people screened, and availability of appointments. The audit took the receptionist 4 hours a week, with 30 minutes a week supervision. The authors report this as a cost-effective approach which resulted in a number of changes, such as better systems for ensuring patient reviews.

Measuring outcome

The outcome of a service is the end result of its intervention on a client or a population, in the short, medium and long terms. One part of the Professional Quality of a service is the quality of outcome from the professional point of view (the providers, referrers such as GPs, and purchasing professionals). In defining Professional Quality standards, each service should reach towards defining quality in terms of outcome and 'health gain', as well as in terms of process, structure and inputs.

One of the best development processes for a group is working together on trying to define what they are aiming to achieve for clients with different conditions. The following suggests ideas for how a group could work towards defining outcome standards of Professional Quality, and methods for measuring performance in relation to these standards (see Chapter 6 for further discussion of standards and measurement).

1 Brainstorm how professionals recognize good and poor quality outcome for a client leaving the service, but also working back and looking at how professionals judge the

outcome of earlier stages (e.g. a treatment session, assessment, etc., depending on the service process). How do professionals in the service judge whether their intervention had the right effect — what do they look for? How do referring professionals judge the quality of outcome of the service? Use these ideas as a basis for discussion about which routine measures to establish.

2 Find out from referring professionals, and professionals advising purchasers, how they judge the quality of outcome of the service. Maintain this debate with regular meetings to discuss progress in developing outcome standards and measures.

3 Define standards of quality outcome before looking for ways to measure and document performance. The tendency is to search for measures and for what can be measured easily, and this can take attention away from what is important.

4 Recognize that general outcome standards and measures are needed which apply to all clients who pass through the service (e.g. a surgical service, GP practice, mental health team), and outcome standards will be needed for the different conditions or diseases the service treats. For example, one outcome measure for all surgical patients is postoperative infection rates, but there are different outcome measures for patients undergoing heart surgery to those undergoing lung surgery.

5 Recognize that outcome is always a matter of judgement: the issue is how to make the judgements better informed (e.g. judgements about the effect of a particular intervention on the client, how to define outcomes, which measures to use, how often, and how to interpret them).

6 Draw from research into outcome measures in general, for the service and for different conditions dealt with by the service. (The King's Fund Quality Abstracts are a good place to start, and they will do a literature search.) Many studies are scientific evaluations of particular treatments or approaches and use methods to assess outcome which are too expensive and elaborate to use routinely (e.g. the Nottingham Health Profile). Many aim to understand causal mechanisms between structure/process and outcome. However, some of these methods can be used for a small sample and suggest ideas.

There is a growing body of research into developing routine outcome measures for quality management, for example a CASPE study of short-term outcomes at Freeman Hospital in Newcastle. It is based on four specialties (general surgery (cholecystectomy), medicine (diabetes), cardiology (angioplasty) and geriatrics), and amongst other things aims to define patient outcomes expected by case type, including expected change in health status.

Most work on routine outcome data has been done in the USA, and is expanding rapidly, not least because of criticism of morbidity and mortality comparisons between hospitals (HCFA 1988). The Rutstein *et al.* (1976) study was one of the first to list medical events that indicate quality problems. This study suggests data that could be gathered on these 'suspicious events' and causes investigated (e.g. death from appendicitis or from metastic cervical cancers).

Below are a few examples of general and specific outcome standards, and of measures and indicators:

In-patient:
- Emergency re-admission within 2 weeks of discharge
- Postoperative infection rates
- Return to operating theatre (for same condition)
- Mortality and morbidity rates

Primary care (from Metcalfe 1989, reported in Roberts 1990):
- Immunization and screening population coverage
- Terminal care symptom control, maintenance of function and acceptance of death
- For management of chronic disease, measures of reversal or stabilization of disease (e.g. coma in diabetes)

Other approaches to professional audit

There is a growing body of reports of audits and research into audit methodology (much of which is usefully summarized in the King's Fund Quality Programme Abstracts). Details of audit in general medical practice are to be found in Marinker (1990), for Surgery in RCP (1989), and for Obstetrics and Gynaecology in RCOG (1990). The Department of Health requirements are outlined in DoH (1989) and DoH (1991).

Each of the above are used not only for medical audit, but for nursing and the therapy professions. Other approaches to audit are reported by Heron (1979) and Øvretveit (1988). Both emphasize professionally derived criteria and objective but supportive feedback.

Heron (1979) (and later Kilty 1979) developed a peer review system for general medical practitioners. It is based on humanistic psychology and counselling principles and is used in educational and other services. The system emphasizes each practitioner identifying their own criteria for improvement and enlisting peers to give them feedback about their performance. The Peer Review Process reported by Øvretveit (1988) was used in a multidisciplinary mental handicap service. The process involved two similar work groups developing their own standards and methods for measuring performance. Each group presented their quality system to the other group and revised it in the light of their feedback. Performance was then measured and improvements made for 3 months before a second peer review, which also included clients. Appendix 5 gives an overview of the process.

Another approach is for professional groups to use quality tools more commonly used in commercial services and manufacturing to establish standards and make improvements. Professional groups have used methods described in this report, such as the flow-process model (Chapter 3) to identify Professional Quality problems and to set standards.

In the quality framework presented in this report, most audit approaches can be used to improve Professional Quality. However, these processes must be linked into other processes for improving Client and Management Quality. Ideally, and in time, each sub-service should move towards establishing a comprehensive set of standards, and a Quality Management Cycle which covers all three dimensions of quality.

Introducing audit

The general conclusion of most research and experience is that changes in behaviour are best achieved by professionals themselves agreeing what needs to be done, and by peer group pressure and recognition. However, systematic audit is rarely introduced voluntarily. In collegial groups it is difficult for one individual to make the proposal or to ensure that all are involved. There is also the time, effort and support necessary to start and then continue audit.

Audit is now a requirement in the UK (DoH 1989, 1991), but there are no requirements about which type of method a service should use. The British model is different from the US model, relying less on sanctions and management control than on education, example and profession direction. Unfortunately many services will accept the current informal and unsystematic methods as audit.

One of the immediate incentives for systematic audit is that it will be important to purchasers' contract decisions, and they know effective audit when they see it. Another is avoiding negligence claims. However, as with quality generally, audit will need to be 'sold' to each professional group (see Chapter 8), their proposals for audit methods sought, and targets agreed for establishing audit.

The following principles help to choose an audit approach, and to develop audit:

1 Start with a simple approach based on the Quality Correction Cycle. That is, one which selects one or a few subjects for audit, and establishes the discipline of setting standards, data gathering, problem–cause analysis and evaluation (Chapter 5). The cycle provides a framework for staff to learn and become familiar with the methods and with a systematic approach. It also allows organizational links to be forged between audit processes and general management, which will not be overloaded by the, usually minor, service changes called for by this type of audit.

2 Develop this approach with more sophisticated methods for selecting subjects, for data gathering and documentation, and for problem–cause analysis. Develop links between audit process and other management processes.

3 Move to more comprehensive audit approach based on the Quality Management Cycle (Chapter 6). Here the service defines a range of Professional Quality features, and establishes a range of standards (rather than just one, or a few for specific subjects). Performance is measured routinely in relation to these standards (e.g. annually for the whole set, monthly for priority standards) and areas are selected for action (using a Quality Correction Cycle).

4 Link or integrate Professional Audit with Quality Management Cycles for Client and Management Quality dimensions. Ideally, establish a full set of standards as discussed in Chapter 6.

The general principle is to phase in quality methods in stages which are compatible with staff abilities and with organizational structure.

Computers and special information are not necessary in order to begin. Existing information such as performance indicators are useful for comparisons between specialties, such as clinical re-attendance and length of in-patient stays. Other information is available from assessment records, referral letters, theatre registers, discharge summaries, and from patient administration systems, and clinical data capture. The Hospital In-Patient Enquiry contains information about discharge and/or death, but there are limitations to the data, not least that they are based on a sample of only 1% of patients (Roberts 1990).

Computers and better records are essential to more sophisticated approaches to audit. Management information systems should be developed to include provision for audit information (e.g. resource management systems). However, even in the early stages professionals must have the necessary resources (extra clerical time and other support) to undertake meaningful audit, as well as help from management to introduce improvements. This is the other side of the bargain that management must strike with professional staff to start and maintain audit.

Summary

- Professional Quality is one of the three dimensions of health service quality.
- It must be considered separately because many aspects of the quality of a health service can only be assessed and improved by professionals. Service Quality, however, is not the sole province of professionals.
- Professional audit undertaken within each profession is the main way of improving Professional Quality, but structures and processes for dealing with inter-professional issues should also be established.
- If the framework described in this report were adopted, Professional Quality standards should be developed and integrated with Client and Management Quality standards in a Quality Management Cycle.

There are four main types of medical audit, many of which are also used by other professions: internal retrospective, external retrospective, concurrent active, and criterion-based audit.

Professional groups should select a method of audit which is suited to their circumstances, and be provided with the necessary resources to undertake meaningful audit. Management should 'sell' the need for audit and ask for proposals from each group. Management have a legitimate interest in audit processes and outcomes: they should agree progress targets, the resources that they will provide, and assist in making changes called for by evidence from audit. Management also need to receive regular reports, to review the cost-effectiveness of the chosen audit method with each professional group, and to ensure that audit links with other quality initiatives.

5
Management Quality

*M*ANY HEALTH SERVICE *managers believe that there is a cost—quality tradeoff: that raising quality will cost more, or that reducing costs means lower quality. In fact higher quality means lower costs because waste, delays and errors are reduced. Quality is not just meeting customer requirements, but also increasing productivity and efficiency and reducing costs. This is achieved by attention to the Management Quality dimension of a service — to designing the service and operating it in the most efficient and productive way.*

Introduction

The third of the three dimensions of quality is the least considered in public health services. In my view it is the most important to the future of the service and central to the quality approach.

Management Quality does not refer directly to the quality of the management of a service, although it is largely determined by the competence of managers. It refers to designing the service and running it without waste, duplication and mistakes. This chapter explains what is meant by Management Quality, and considers how it is measured. It looks at the cost of poor Management Quality and describes tools and methods which staff can use to improve the quality of all three dimensions of a health service.

What is the Management Quality of a service?

Some theorists view quality as customer satisfaction. They see productivity as something different, which sometimes conflicts with customer satisfaction and hence quality. For example, Denton (1989) argues that it is short-sighted to make productivity a higher priority than quality, which he defines as customer service. He proposes the concept of 'qualitivity' to emphasize their equal priority.

In contrast, the general definition of quality in this book is something which encompasses both customer satisfaction and productivity. That aspect of quality which relates to productivity is defined as Management Quality.

Management Quality

The selection and deployment of resources in the most efficient way to meet customer needs, within limits and directives.

One reason for looking at Management Quality separately is to show more clearly how quality improvements save money *and* increase productivity (Fig. 5.1). In the past, cost savings were made in health services in ways which reduced productivity. Not recruiting clerks throws administration on to expensive professionals. Making do with equipment that breaks down or is not suitable is a false economy in the long term. Freezing posts leads to staff trying to deal with the extra work, and going off sick and exhausted or leaving the service, which leads to extra costs to recruit and train new staff.

Cost savings made in this way are not the only possible response to funding crises. They are symptomatic of a more widespread attitude which is not confined to public services. In commercial services in the West, short-term thinking arises because of financing structures and fear of take-overs. In health services there have been few short-term savings which have not incurred considerable costs in the long term. Under-investment has produced many inefficiencies and accounts for some of the unnecessarily high cost of some services.

Poor Management Quality

To understand what Management Quality is about in practical terms, think back over your last week at work. Consider how much time you spent chasing someone who did not call back, or trying to get information which someone should have supplied. Add to this any time wasted doing the wrong work because you were given the wrong information, or because it was not clear what was wanted. Add delays caused by waiting for the information, or for supplies you were promised. How much needless extra time did you

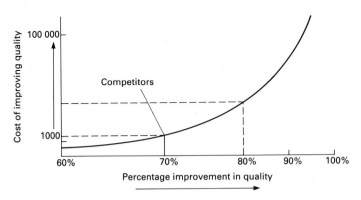

Fig. 5.1 Relate investment in quality to the market sector. Investment in quality always pays off in the long term but quality improvements get more expensive. Thus the rate, amount and subjects for investment depend in part on computer performance.

spend trying to find something in the filing system or stores, or did you not bother to look because you knew you would never find it? Then add work which someone else was also doing which you duplicated, or work which will never be used, or which no one knows why it is done, or which no one would notice if it were not done. Add time complying with procedures which are no longer necessary, or working with or training someone in unnecessarily complex procedures which are difficult for the experts to get right every time.

Add also, the time dealing with angry clients who have been mistreated by the service, or dealing with complaints which could easily have been avoided, or re-doing work which was done wrongly. Then add time for double-checking things which you are not sure are done correctly.

All this time can be estimated, but another aspect of poor quality is difficult to quantify. This stems from your creativity and productivity simply being ground down by it all. It is the effect on your motivation and morale of all the time-wasting and things that go wrong and which you do not even notice any more because 'it's just how things are'.

The cumulative effect of poor quality is insidious — it accounts for much of the 'why bother' mentality and indifference. This attitude becomes understandable as a necessary survival strategy — it is an insult to suggest that some people will never care about their work. Across the organization it is possible to begin to quantify the cost of a poor quality workplace and frustrating work, in terms of absenteeism and high turnover and the high cost of replacing staff — if you can get them.

Cost of poor quality

The costs of not doing the right thing, right first time

Making good

- Time spent dealing with needless complaints
- Legal costs of defending negligence claims
- Cost of claims (and higher insurance)
- 'Re-work' (e.g. re-admissions due to poor quality assessments or treatments, returned supplies or services)

Poor supplies and services

- Delays waiting for supplies and information
- Wrong supplies and information ('making do' costs, re-ordering costs)

Poor process quality

- Giving suppliers inaccurate orders
- Doing the wrong work because of poor assessment of clients' wants and needs
- Doing the wrong work because given the wrong information
- Over-complex procedures and high cost of coordination
- Any rule or procedure which does not contribute to quality
- Duplication
- Mistakes and waste due to poor recruitment, training or staff lack of knowledge of the service process

Difficult to quantify (but highest cost)

- Bad reputation, lost referrals
- Corrosive effect of poor qualities on staff (loss of motivation, poor morale, staff dissatisfaction, lack of creativity and innovation, absenteeism, high turnover, high recruitment and training costs)

This is all without adding the costs of materials which were thrown away, or never used because they were the wrong order, or supplied but never ordered. The total costs in terms of wasted time and wasted material is the cost of poor quality. Some of it is other people's fault and some of it is your fault, even if you went wrong in assuming that someone else would do their work correctly, or do what they said they would.

Across the organization the total cost is likely to be 25–45% of operating costs. That is without adding the highest cost — the human cost in terms of poor morale and motivation and the loss of staff initiative and energy. This is not eastern Europe, it is where you work.

Reversing the poor quality spiral — the human costs

Figure 5.2 represents the self-reinforcing cycle or upward spiral which quality programmes aim to establish and sustain.

Staff often feel that their work is as pointless as digging a hole and then being made to fill it in. Sometimes worse — being made to dig a hole with a useless spade, in a way that they know is the wrong way, and in gravel which just slips back before they can throw it out of the hole. They are not even allowed the satisfaction of digging a decent hole and filling it in properly!

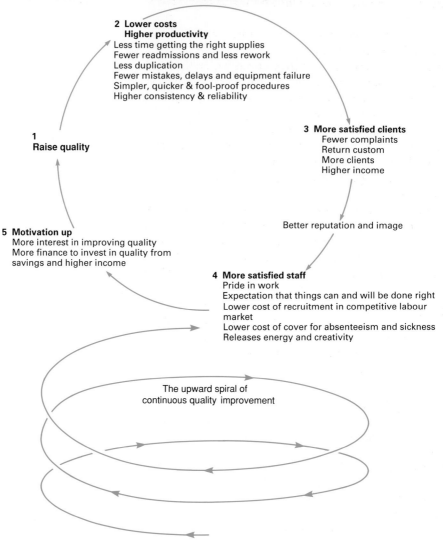

Fewer negligence claims, less legal and insurance costs
Less time dealing with complaints

2 Lower costs
  Higher productivity
Less time getting the right supplies
Fewer readmissions and less rework
Less duplication
Fewer mistakes, delays and equipment failure
Simpler, quicker & fool-proof procedures
Higher consistency & reliability

1
Raise quality

3 More satisfied clients
  Fewer complaints
  Return custom
  More clients
  Higher income

Better reputation and image

5 Motivation up
More interest in improving quality
More finance to invest in quality from
savings and higher income

4 More satisfied staff
  Pride in work
  Expectation that things can and will be done right
  Lower cost of recruitment in competitive labour
  market
  Lower cost of cover for absenteeism and sickness
  Releases energy and creativity

The upward spiral of
continuous quality improvement

Fig. 5.2 Raising quality reduces costs and increases productivity and income.

The real benefits of improving Management Quality come from the effect of the improvements on staff. The end result is to make work more satisfying and less frustrating because staff do not waste effort making up for the things that keep going wrong. But just as important is the effect on staff of their being able to take control of their work processes and themselves eliminate one by one, and once and for all, the causes of the errors, time-wasting and delays.

People want to work in a satisfying environment where they can get on with the job and perform their best. By improving Management Quality they can avoid waste and frustration, and they can give clients a better service and be thought of as competent, rather than having to apologize for delays or mistakes.

People will not take more pride in their work because they are told to, but because they are given control and methods which work. The positive effects on staff of improving quality only occur when they have been involved in analysing and resolving Management Quality problems. If staff are trained to do this and are viewed as experts in the process, and if they are given the power to overcome their problems, they then begin to take the initiative and feel that they can do something about their service. They assume responsibility and feel valued — the opposite of what often happens now.

I believe that these changes are essential to the future of health services, but they will not come from frightening staff about employment prospects or for failing to meet arbitrary standards, nor from exhortation and 'cheer-leader' performances. The changes will only come by properly equipping staff with proven tools which enable them to analyse their process and its problems. They will only come by giving staff the power to make the changes, and by managers changing their role to enable staff to make these changes. The rest of this book describes these tools and considers how to achieve this.

Management quality

- One of the three dimensions of the quality of a health service
- Considered as a separate dimension because only some of the inefficiencies of the service process are uncovered by examining Client and Professional Quality dimensions
- Measured by estimating the cost of poor quality
- Most quality costs can be quantified and most are avoidable
- Improving the Management Quality of the service means enabling staff continually to eliminate causes of mistakes, duplication, and waste — it is about ensuring that the right things are done right, first time, every time
- Improvements to Management Quality also lead to improvements in Client Quality and Professional Quality — resources are freed and delays and mistakes are reduced for clients
- Cost reductions and efficiency savings are not made at the expense of customer service, at least not when these savings are made as part of a quality approach

Improving Management Quality

Improvements to the Management Quality of the service are made by ensuring proper *design* of the service delivery process for the function it is to serve, and proper *operation* of the service delivery process — ensuring that the different elements of the right staff, materials, clients and information are brought together in the right places in the right time and in the right way.

As implied above, the Management Quality of the service at any time is measured by costing the extra time and materials and other costs incurred when things are not done correctly the first time. Waiting times and delays are also an indicator of Management Quality. This is because anything preventing a fast response is usually a weakness in the service process, often a bottleneck due to inadequate capacity at the next stage, or because supplies and information are inefficient.

The quality approach aims to resolve these problems once and for all through a Quality Correction Cycle using systematic methods to discover and deal with the root cause. It is based on evidence that the cost of accepting or ignoring poor quality is always higher than the cost of resolving the problem.

How then should managers and staff go about improving the Management Quality of their service? There are three ingredients — a motive (encouraged by the right service culture), an opportunity (time and support for staff), and a weapon (quality methods). This and the next chapter consider the methods — the 'technical' side of quality. Chapter 8 considers motive and opportunity and the 'people' side of quality.

Improving Management Quality

A Motive: the culture of the service must be one in which staff wish to make improvements (Chapter 8)
An Opportunity: staff need the training, support, and time to use the methods (Chapter 8)
A Weapon: the tools of quality — quality methods and concepts (this chapter and Chapter 6)

Most of the pressures on managers are to manage quantity and costs — to increase output and reduce costs immediately. Managers and purchasers need to understand the current cost–quantity–quality relationship in the service and agree what balance to strike. It is then possible to look at how quality can be improved without increasing costs. This is done by identifying and costing quality problems, and then removing them once and for all. The following describes methods for doing this. The rest of this chapter and the next consider quality methods and tools. Some of these were introduced in previous chapters: methods for measuring client satisfaction, the Quality Correction Cycle, and the Quality Management Cycle.

Quality tools and methods

There is nothing mysterious or difficult about quality tools and methods. They are simply ways for systematically identifying, analysing and resolving the most costly quality problems. These methods have proved their worth in a range of organizations, and are now being applied and developed in health services, especially in the USA (McLaughlin & Kaluzny 1990, NDT 1991). Although training and time to apply the methods are essential, high levels of skill or ability are not needed to learn and apply the methods with benefit.

Quality tools and methods

Substance not style — exhortation and charm schools do not resolve quality problems. Give staff proven and effective tools to identify quality problems and to resolve root causes once and for all.
- Tools for process design and redesign (p. 84, and Chapter 3)
- Methods for estimating quality costs (p. 85)
- A framework for removing root causes of quality problems (the Quality Correction Cycle, p. 87)
- Tools for picking out the most costly quality problems (p. 86)
- Methods for detecting causes of problems (p. 87)
- A framework for continuous quality improvement (the Quality Management Cycle — Chapter 6)
- Methods for setting standards and specification (Chapter 6)
- Measurement methods (Chapter 6)
- Methods for listing causes of quality problems (p. 87)
- Methods for gathering and analysing data to find the main causes of quality problems (Chapter 6)
- Methods for involving staff in making quality improvements (Chapter 8)
- Methods for statistical process control (Chapter 6)

Tools for service process design

One set of tools helps to build in quality by designing processes for the simplest and fastest flow. This does not mean an architect's plan, although the physical movements of staff, clients and materials are important. Neither does it mean a computer system's diagram of information flows. Rather, it is about designing the service as a process, focusing on the client's movements, and on what is done to and for the client at different stages. The physical layout and information flows should be based on this 'service process'.

Service process design

Service process design maps the flow of clients to and through the service to work out the simplest and fastest ways of bringing staff, clients, information, equipment, and other materials together in the right way at the right times.

Redesign involves mapping what happens at present, and working out simpler, faster and more efficient ways of carrying through the process.

Prerequisites are to be clear about who the service is for and what it aims to achieve for these clients (Chapters 2 and 3).

There are few health services which are set up by thinking beforehand about how different types of clients are to be handled, from their entry to the service to their exit. Sophisticated design methods include 'blueprinting' (Shostack 1984), and Just-in-Time methodology to reduce waiting times and inventory costs, streamline processes, and continually highlight quality problems.

The Management Quality of all services can be improved by redesigning the service process. This means redesigning the primary client process, as well as the sub-processes carried out within each stage. Most services can start by modelling the service using the flow-process framework described in Chapter 3. The framework was used there to consider the process purely in terms of the situations which affected client perceptions. The same framework should be used to highlight where mistakes and waste occur. From this a list of Management Quality problems is produced. This will immediately suggest better ways of organizing the process to simplify it and to avoid mistakes and waste. The sections below describe methods for deciding which problems to tackle and how to remove them once and for all.

In my experience, staff are pleased to analyse their service process using this framework and are helped by this structured approach. However, there are limits to the redesign that they can tackle. Over-complex processes are often a result of trying to meet the needs of too many different types of clients with a single process. It becomes necessary to devise separate processes for different types of clients, or reduce the range of clients served, both of which are strategic quality issues (Chapter 2) rather than operational redesign.

Methods for costing poor Management Quality

A second set of methods is for quantifying the current cost of poor Management Quality. Calculating this cost is the first step towards making improvements.

The total cost of poor quality is more than the cost of poor Management Quality. The total costs include the costs incurred through poor Client Quality discussed in Chapter 3, such as lost custom and complaints (referred to below as 'external failure costs').

Many commercial companies have routine reports of current quality costs, which are scrutinized and treated as seriously as other financial and sales reports. Poor Management Quality costs can be calculated in different ways. Crosby (1979) provides accessible and useful guidance. The commonest way in the UK is to divide quality costs into four categories.

1 *Prevention costs*: the cost of any action taken to investigate, prevent or reduce defects and failures (e.g. cost of time in quality circles, quality training, salaries of quality specialists).
2 *Appraisal/assurance costs*: the costs of assessing the quality achieved (e.g. cost of time spent monitoring specifications, getting client feedback).
3 *Internal failure costs*: the costs arising from the failure to achieve the quality specified before the client leaves the service (e.g. information from referrers not available, pre-operative tests incomplete).

Quality costing

- Gives an idea of the relative size of each problem and the potential savings
- Makes it possible to compare problems to decide which to address
- Helps judge and track the impact and cost-effectiveness of different changes
- Estimation should not be avoided because accurate information is not available

---

4 *External failure costs*: the costs arising from failure to achieve the quality specified after the client has received the service (e.g. time spent dealing with complaints, readmission due to inadequate treatment or assessment).

My own research found difficulties in assigning costs to these categories. For example, is the time spent redesigning a client questionnaire a prevention or an appraisal cost? Each service will need to work out how to apply these categories. This is one reason for caution when comparing quality costs between departments or services who may not use the categories in the same way.

Other difficulties are how to deal with overheads, and obtaining accurate figures and cooperation from overloaded finance departments. Often this is not necessary as precise figures are not needed in the early stages. Although an estimation of quality costs should never be avoided because accurate figures are not available, it is important that the estimates have credibility, especially if major investments are contemplated, or to set cost reduction targets. Crosby's comment that early estimates are one-third of the real costs are borne out in my experience.

Identifying priority problems

The following describes one way of costing poor Management Quality. The approach was developed to raise staff awareness of costs and to help prioritize problems. The first step is to represent the service process using the service flow-process framework described in Chapter 3. This model is then used to identify points in the process and situations where things go wrong, or where materials or time are wasted. These are defined as Management Quality problems.

The cost of each problem is then calculated in terms of the staff time taken up, or the wasted materials, or any other waste. Usually rough estimates are all that is needed. The assumptions are that the process could be operated perfectly; that when it does not work perfectly there is waste, and that this waste can be costed.

After calculating the cost to the service of each Management Quality problem it is possible to consider the cost of resolving the problem and the rate of return on investment. Each problem is considered in turn and an estimate made of how much it would take to eliminate the problem once and for all, or the cost of drastically reducing the severity of the problem. It is sometimes difficult to do this without a full problem–cause analysis (see below) but usually an estimate is possible to decide which problems to look at in detail.

This approach to costing quality gives a list of the quality problems, their cost and the cost of elimination (or problem-reduction). Any group can work through this process in less than 2 hours and propose practical improvements which produce considerable savings.

The next step is to pick out a quality problem to work on, to prioritize quality problems for correction. There are a number of things to consider. First, the costings will show the few problems that cost the service the most. A rule of thumb is that 20% of the problems incur 80% of the costs of poor quality, but the most costly problems are not necessarily the best to start with. Some are extremely expensive to resolve. More important are the savings which can be made with respect to the investment. Resolving a smaller problem may well produce a greater return on investment.

However, in the early stages of a quality programme, cost savings are not the only consideration. It is just as important to select a problem that is relatively easy for staff to resolve, in order to build up their confidence and experience with the methods. It is also important to rate each problem in terms of which cause the most aggravation for staff.

Considerations in prioritizing quality problems for correction:
- Which problems cost the service the most?
- Which problems cost the least to solve in relation to the savings? (i.e. produce the highest return on investment)
- Which problems are easy for staff to solve, and make work less frustrating for them?

The Quality Correction Cycle

The Quality Correction Cycle is not a method, but a framework for using methods. It a systematic way of working on a quality problem to resolve it once and for all. Services sometimes use quality methods, but not in a methodical way. They might pick out the main quality problems, but do not properly resolve the problems or use ineffective or costly methods to do so. The Quality Correction Cycle deploys quality methods in a structured way to deal with problems. The last chapter showed that many approaches to audit are based on the principles of this cycle.

Figure 5.3 shows the main parts of the cycle and then considers the methods used in each part of the cycle.

Problem – cause analysis

After selecting the priority problem to be addressed, the aim is to follow the Quality Correction Cycle to analyse the problem to discover the cause, and to take steps to make sure the problem does not happen again. There are different methods for problem–cause analysis, all based on the principles of systematic analysis and data gathering. Untrained staff groups do not naturally take a systematic approach. They tend to fly into speculations about solutions without stating the problem properly, or define problems only in terms of assumed causes. This can lead to wasting time and money on changing the wrong things.

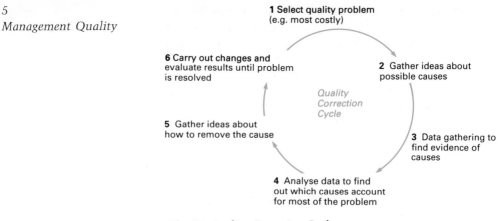

Fig. 5.3 Quality Correction Cycle.

A simple approach for a staff group to use is as follows. Having defined and selected the problem, using methods already described, the group considers possible causes (part 2 of the cycle shown in Fig. 5.3). A simple method for doing this is to use an Ishikawa 'fishbone' diagram (Ishikawa 1985). This helps to gather hypotheses about causes before seeking out evidence.

As an illustration, take the problem of missing or incomplete patient notes for follow-up appointments. A flip-chart diagram is made with the quality problem on the right as the 'fish head'. The 'bones' of the diagram joining the 'spine' list all possible causes. Staff suggest causes under the headings of personnel, procedures, equipment, materials, information and 'other.' The next step is to decide what evidence would be needed to establish whether a suspected cause was indeed the real cause (part 3 of the cycle).

Members of the group are delegated to gather the necessary evidence, which is then analysed and represented using a Pareto diagram (Hutchins 1990). This shows which causes had the greatest influence on the effect (i.e. lost patient notes — part 4 of the cycle). The Pareto rule of thumb is that a few causes account for 80% of the effect.

Once the main causes are discovered in this way, a plan is made to remove the causes of the problem (part 5 of the cycle). Progress is measured by regularly monitoring the number of lost notes. In some cases the cost of problem elimination or reduction is estimated, in order to obtain authorization for investment finance to remove the causes.

The point of using these methods and the correction cycle is to ensure that the problem is resolved before moving onto the next problem. Some services make considerable improvements using these methods, especially as part of a quality circle framework (Hutchins 1990).

More sophisticated statistical methods to analyse quality problems will be discussed in the next chapter (statistical process control methods). Not all quality problems need such a thorough approach, but the principle of resolving the problem once and for all must be followed. It is the 'make do' and partial solutions, with the problem recurring, that are so frustrating to staff.

Summary

The simple methods above were presented as methods to improve the Management Quality dimension of a service. However, they are also used to correct problems in Client and Professional Quality.

The next chapter brings together each of the three dimensions of quality in the Quality Management Cycle. It shows how a service would establish a comprehensive set of standards, and make changes which improve all dimensions of the quality of the service.

Management Quality is about:
• Designing the simplest and most efficient combination and flow of the elements needed to meet clients' needs
• Identifying and avoiding problems which cause delays, mistakes, and waste
• Increasing productivity at the same time as cutting costs

Management Quality is measured by calculating the cost of poor quality (the cost consequences of things which are not done correctly the first time). It is improved by costing and removing quality problems once and for all, using a Quality Correction Cycle. The cycle uses proven quality methods, such as process-flow analysis, problem–cause analysis, graphs, and control charts.

Improving Management Quality
• Produces cost savings and better customer service
• Reduces staff frustrations, and makes work more satisfying
• Releases energy and creativity

6

Managing and Controlling Quality

THE AIM OF quality management is not to meet performance standards, nor is it to deal with quality problems. It is to help everyone in the service to take responsibility for controlling quality and to enable them to use quality methods to improve the processes for delivering the service. To have the maximum effect, these methods should be used as part of a Quality Management Cycle.

Introduction

This chapter begins by describing the Quality Management Cycle, which is a framework for using quality methods. Managers need to help staff to learn and use these simple methods, and to become familiar with the cyclical approach and the principle of continuous improvement.

The chapter pays particular attention to the specification and measurement aspects of the Quality Management Cycle. Standards and measurement are often misused and frequently become ends in themselves. They are often introduced in the wrong way and turn already overloaded staff against a quality approach. Quality is then seen only as more procedures and a threatening, punitive set of performance measures. Specification and measurement should be used to help people to focus on the most important things, to understand the effects of their actions, and to communicate clearly about what is happening or is intended to happen.

The difficulties are not in deciding how to specify or measure something, but in deciding what to specify and measure, and who does it. The chapter proposes that the subjects be selected according to the quality problems faced by the service, and according to the stage of evolution of the quality programme in the service. It shows how to set standards for and measure each of the three dimensions of health service quality (Client, Professional and Management Quality) and how to ensure an integrated comprehensive set of standards appropriate to the stage of quality sophistication of a service. It assumes that a service wishes to use these methods to develop a quality system for continuous improvement, rather than only to comply with externally imposed specifications or standards (Chapter 7), which should always be viewed as a minimum requirement.

The chapter finishes with a discussion of statistical process control and of the philosophy of continuous process improvement underpinning the use of this methodology. Through this discussion of quality methods, the chapter also explains more about the philosophy of quality, and the change in staff attitudes and the role and relationships of managers that is necessary to manage quality.

The Quality Management Cycle

Earlier chapters considered how to identify the target clients of the service and their needs. This chapter focuses on the operational management of the service, and on how the data from the business strategy are used as a starting point in the Quality Management Cycle (Fig. 6.1).

The following first summarises the main parts of the cycle and then discusses in detail the methods used in each part of the cycle.

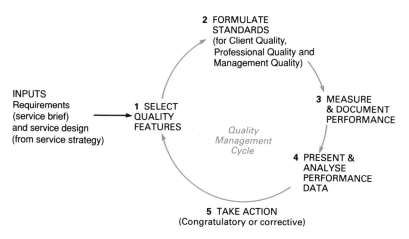

Fig. 6.1 The Quality Management Cycle.

Inputs from service strategy

Many of the quality features that are the start of the cycle come from market analyses and from quality specifications in purchaser contracts. This links issues of strategy to the operational Quality Management Cycle.

Background data — requirements

These data from service strategy define what is critical to attract clients to the service, and the things that influence purchaser decisions (some of which are already defined in contracts). This information should be available in order to select the quality features in the first part of the cycle. The aim is to improve those features of quality which are important to market performance.

Background data — service design specification

This is the description of the service package/concept, and flow-process diagrams of the service delivery process (Chapter 3).

1 Select quality features

Quality features are definitions of those aspects of service
which are critical to each dimension of service quality at a
particular time (e.g. a Client Quality feature may be waiting
time, a Professional Quality feature may be how well assessments are performed, and a Management Quality feature
may be clients failing to attend appointments).

A service will choose quality features in a way which
when it first introduces a quality programme is different to
later stages. At the start only a few will be picked out so
that the full cycle can be established. Too many features
makes it impossible to set standards, measure performance
and follow through the cycle to action for all the quality
features. It shows the service is not clear about priorities
and has not done a strategic analysis.

2 Formulate standards

In this part of the cycle, a service takes each quality feature
and formulates a standard for it. Standards are formulated
for Client, Professional, and Management Quality features,
and brought together to create an integrated and balanced
set of standards for the service. In doing this the service
addresses any conflicts between standards, and picks out
areas where changes may improve all dimensions of quality
at the same time.

3 Measure and document performance

Once the service has standards, it is then possible to measure
performance in relation to each standard. All can then see if
what was intended is in fact happening. In this part of the
cycle, staff who were involved in formulating the standards
collect and record performance against standards, using the
chosen measures or indicators. They use sampling methodology to decide representative samples to record, and simple
check sheets and other recording methods to document
performance.

4 Analyse and present performance

The records are used to analyse and present performance.
Performance is not presented in terms of averages, or highest
and lowest, or as lists of figures, but in terms of graphs and
charts that show the variations in performance for each
item specified and measured. These are posted or made
available to all staff, and can easily be understood. Only a
few standards are measured and reported frequently.

In time, the service will develop a wider set of standards. Decisions then have to be made about which to measure and report frequently and which to measure on a longer term basis. Different performances will need to be measured and reported daily, weekly, monthly, quarterly or annually.

5 Action

The point of setting standards and measuring performance is to take action: either congratulatory or corrective action. All the earlier effort selecting important features and measuring performance is wasted if staff are not congratulated, or action is not taken to improve performance. Corrective action may be simple or it may need a more sustained approach using the Quality Correction Cycle described in the last chapter.

6 Reassessment

Once quality performance is stable and standards are being met, the cycle then returns to the quality features part (part 1). The service reassesses whether to continue to improve performance on the original quality features (by raising standards), or whether to add new quality features. The purpose of the cycle is to ensure that the quality methods are used in the right way and in the right sequence, but also to ensure that the service has a process for continuously improving quality.

Phasing in quality

Different methods are used when a service first begins the cycle. At the early stages, a service will pick a few quality features from an analysis of the most serious quality problems. The key here is to establish the cycle, not to have a full set of standards. Below it is suggested that the flow-process analysis is used to choose quality features early on.

As more data become available from market research and business strategy, these can be fed into the part of the cycle concerned with selecting quality features, and the cycle can take in more areas of the service.

Before looking at the methods used in each part of the cycle, it is important to understand the differences between the traditional management process and the Quality Management Cycle. Why is such an elaborate approach needed to manage quality? Surely there are less expensive ways of meeting purchaser's quality requirements? Surely all this costs more than it saves?

*Differences between traditional management process and
the Quality Management Cycle*

The Quality Management Cycle shows some similarities to classic 'rational management' as outlined in introductions to management. Indeed some managers understand the Quality Management Cycle in these terms, as a version of management-by-objectives with a few quality standards. They think they know what is required of the service and what clients want, and they decide the most important things to specify, to make it clear to staff what to concentrate on. They make sure that staff know their instructions, they measure performance against these specifications, and take action where performance is not up to standard, and may even revise specifications upwards. They assume that managing quality is therefore similar to what good managers (or those who follow the texts) have always done — just more of the same. But if this is so, why do managers find it so difficult to make significant improvements to quality using traditional management approaches?

In some services, traditional management approaches, applied conscientiously, do raise quality for a while. Simply making clear what is expected of staff, measuring performance and taking action often does improve all dimensions of quality. Indeed, in one service a first step in establishing a Quality Management Cycle was to clarify aims and responsibilities (Øvretveit 1990), and it is proposed later that this is the starting point where these organizational fundamentals are not clear.

Why traditional management has a limited impact on quality

The impact of traditional management approaches diminishes and does not produce continual quality improvements. It is not the obvious mistakes that explain this, such as too many standards and specifications, complicated and inaccurate measures, staff not following the manager's instructions.

Neither is it because the starting statement of quality features is wrong. For example, managers making assumptions about client needs, or not including Professional and Management Quality features, or not knowing what is critical to market performance. Rather it is because managers do not use the two key ingredients:

• Quality methods (for specifying, measuring and controlling quality), and
• Enabling staff to take responsibility for managing

quality and to take part in the Quality Management Cycle

Not only do they misunderstand the quality philosophy, but they give staff the wrong understanding of what quality is about. They miss the opportunity to convey this philosophy in the way they introduce a quality programme, and by changing the way in which they work with their staff.

The Quality Management Cycle is often introduced as part of existing ineffective management processes, and fitted into a traditional hierarchical and bureaucratic structure. The cycle describes what needs to be done, not who does it. Just as important as using specifications and measurement methods within the cycle is involving the right people in formulating the specifications, in gathering the measurement data, and in carrying out the control actions.

The methods lose their power if staff do not take part enthusiastically. Staff must understand how these methods help them and the service to improve quality. They must be motivated, with the time, training and support to use the methods. Although this is not easy to arrange (see Chapter 8), the risk is that without such organizational and cultural changes, quality methods will reinforce the ineffective bureaucratic patterns, working relations and power structures in the service.

Middle managers are the key to a quality strategy. One of the most difficult decisions they face in the early stages is how to get started. At the one extreme they can superimpose quality methods onto the current management process. At the other extreme they can go all-out to introduce a rapid and comprehensive change in working methods and in organizational structure and relations. I would argue for a gradual phased introduction, which I believe is the most realistic for most NHS providers.

There are risks and opportunity costs. Managers must make up their minds about what is possible in their service and how to 'pace' quality. The discussion below of different methods to be used within each part of the cycle aims to help these decisions. It tries to convey an idea of the differences between current management practice and basic, as well as more sophisticated, quality approaches.

Differences between the Quality Management Cycle and traditional management

1 *Staff responsibility*
Staff take part in all phases of the cycle: in selecting

95

quality features, formulating standards, in deciding measurement and recording methods, in sampling, measuring and recording, in analysis and presentation, and in taking corrective action.

2 *Focus on processes*
Staff deepen their understanding of how their service process operates. In the early stages they draw a process-flow diagram, and in later stages they use control charts to identify critical variations.

3 *Continuous improvement*
The methods automatically direct attention to the most important things and to continual improvement, not just to meeting minimum standards. Standards are interim targets on the way to an ideal. The assumption is that the current standard will be revised upwards.

4 *Intrinsic incentives*
The incentives to make continual improvements are *intrinsic* to the process and the work. Satisfaction comes from taking responsibility and from learning and using powerful tools, and making visible improvements, not from avoiding punishment or from external material rewards.

5 *Reduce variations*
Working to reduce the variation in the process automatically and continually improves average performance.

Quality methods within the cycle

The following assumes that the groundwork has been done: that the service has a strategy, has defined its target clients and their needs, and is clear about the requirements that it has to meet and the overall service design. In addition, it assumes that this information is available to the people selecting quality features in the first part of the cycle.

The chapter now discusses the methods used in each part of the cycle in more detail. We start with how to select the key quality features of a service at a particular time. This the first step in the process of specification. Specification is used by a purchaser to define what they expect of a provider, and by a provider to define what staff need to do. For example,

'all first outpatient appointments for non-urgent con-sultations will be less than 6 weeks from receipt of referral', and, 'all care plans to be discussed with and

agreed by the client', or, 'client waiting times for consultation in outpatients will be less than 1 hour'.

The purpose of specification is to get an unambiguous
statement of what should be happening. Specifications are
procedures, protocols and policies, but we will here concentrate on specification in terms of standards. Shortly we will
consider different views about what is meant by a standard,
about how to tell a good from a bad standard, and about how
standards should be formulated and used.

Cycle Part 1: Selecting key quality features

Quality features are those aspects of a service which are
critical to quality and which need to be specified, measured
and controlled to assure quality. A service would define
many features of each of the Client, Professional, and Management Quality dimensions, but would only select a few to
specify as standards for frequent measurement. Many of the
mistakes in the next part of the cycle (formulating standards)
arise from not being selective in deciding what to concentrate
on. If specification is not to become a bureaucratic exercise,
then it is important to select and focus on the most important
aspects of a service for control or improvement at a particular time. As these specifications become established and as
performance improves, other things will be specified.

A service selects only a few of the most important features
for the Quality Management Cycle when it first begins a
quality programme. To start with it is only possible to set
standards for a few features, and measure performance and
take action for these. It is more important to follow through
and establish the cycle, than to try to measure performance
and take action on all standards.

At the start, quality features are defined in terms of the
most serious quality problems of the service, which are
revealed by process-flow analyses and/or market research.
Later the service draws upon market research data to define
a more extensive set of quality features. Decisions are then
made about which standards should be measured routinely
and which less frequently.

Selecting quality features and specifying in terms of standards is a waste of time if the service has not specified basic
aspects of organization. Some quality programmes are
launched into a service where people are not clear about
their responsibilities or the objectives and priorities of the
service. The programme fails because the basic organizational
infrastructure is not there to support it (see Chapter 8).
Action is not taken because it is not clear who is responsible,
or, if it is, they have no authority.

In due course, a service will move into a more sophisticated phase to control quality through prevention, and to control the quality of processes. In this phase of true quality assurance, many quality features are decided from input and process models, and specifications are established in terms of upper and lower limits from process control charts.

Each service must work out which are the key things to specify in relation to Client, Professional and Management Quality at a particular time. The following gives some guidance as to how to select quality features when developing a quality system.

Summary: Select quality features according to the problems and level of quality sophistication of the service

A service must have clearly defined organization to be able to carry out a Quality Management Cycle. Once the basics of organization are specified, the service can move on to defining, measuring and improving quality.

Phase 1: quality features are the outstanding quality problems

To start with, the focus is on completely removing the most outstanding quality problems. This is to take the first step away from fire-fighting towards prevention. In this phase the purpose of specification is to help overcome these problems.

The outstanding quality problems are clarified from discussions with purchasers, market analyses, and from flow-process analyses. The process is analysed from each of the Client, Professional and Management Quality perspectives using process-flow charts. From this the key quality problems are listed and prioritized using quality costing methods.

A decision is then made about the few quality features to be taken forward for the standard-setting phase of the Quality Management Cycle. Performance in relation to these standards is measured. This then makes it possible to judge the effectiveness of actions taken to resolve these key quality problems. For some problems a Quality Correction Cycle will be needed.

Phase 2: extend list of quality features

Once the cycle is established and the most pressing quality problems are overcome, the list of quality features for the cycle can be extended. This involves compiling a list of quality features from the business

---

strategy and market research data. It also involves acknowledging and refining the quality features that are implicit in everyday work (often termed 'standards' by staff), and are implicit in procedures and explicit in professional codes. Decisions are made about which standards to measure routinely, and which to measure less frequently.

Phase 3: specification to control variation

This more sophisticated phase moves into prevention. Specification in this phase focuses on the things that vary, and which, if they are not controlled within a certain range, will threaten quality. Specification subjects are selected by analysing inputs and process to identify critical variables. Specification is in terms of upper and lower control limits (see below).

Because specification is such an expensive and potentially powerful tool, it should be used selectively. Specify those things that are most important for assuring and improving quality at a particular time. Introduce the specification methods and disciplines gradually and in ways in which the purpose and benefits are clear.

Cycle Part 2: Specification and standards

Standards are sometimes specified at different levels of abstraction, even within a single service, and this can cause problems. Statements that are measurable and specified in behavioural terms are essential for quality. A basic skill for managers and staff is to be able to formulate such statements, and to use them.

Standard statements

If we compare examples of standards, we see that, amongst other things, the statements differ in their level of abstraction. Some examples of cleaning standards are:
A 'A high level of cleanliness to be maintained at all times'
B 'The bedded area to be maintained so that no appreciable accumulation of dirt or dust is evident after cleaning'
C 'All surfaces free from dust smears and film, no excess dampness streaking or residual dirt after damp mopping, and no scuff marks or residual dirt after floor scrubbing, as judged on a rating scale by the assessor everyday within 3 hours of cleaning'

The terminology used in this book calls the specific statement a 'standard' (e.g. statement C in the example) and calls the more abstract statement a quality feature (in the example, statement A).

Sometimes people call the specific statements 'criteria', and the more abstract statements 'standards', which is the reverse of the terminology used in this book. For example Wilson (1987) relates specific statements to higher-level statements of objectives and mission. Following the standards for accreditation of Canadian health care, he defines standards simply as 'expectations or requirements', and the more specific statements as 'criteria', defined as 'measurable aspects of desired performance'. For Wilson, criteria 'offer measurable statements by which a product or service can be judged to have met the standard set'.

> **Standard**
>
> A standard is a specific expectation of staff, described in terms of an activity or outcome against which their actions can be measured. The expectation is specified in terms of a level of performance to be achieved on a defined measure or indicator.

The important thing is to recognize that statements of different levels of abstraction are needed, and for all to be clear what is meant by a standard. In the discussion below of steps for setting standards, a standard is the specific statement, and quality feature the more abstract.

Another way of understanding what we mean by a standard is to distinguish it from an objective, or a procedure or policy, with which standards are often confused. Policies usually contain implicit or explicit quality features (which some would call standards) but the statements are too abstract to serve as standards in the sense used here. Operating policies also contain implicit or explicit standards. They provide one set of ready-made standards that a service should identify and list with other potential standards before choosing and formulating a full set.

> *What is the difference between a standard and an objective, a policy or a procedure?*
>
> An objective gives direction by defining a goal or end to be reached, after which the objective has been achieved. In contrast, standards apply all the time, or are revised less frequently than objectives.
> For example, a person has as an objective to reach

London by 10 a.m. They also have certain standards of travel which apply all the time and which they will not compromise (comfort, convenience, safety etc.). Usually the standards come first and define how they will reach the objective: they will redefine the objective (10.30 a.m.) rather than change standards. But sometimes the objective is so important to them that they redefine the standards.

How do you tell a 'good' from a 'bad' standard?

If a standard is to be of use it should be:
- *Measurable*. Standards in the framework reported here are defined in terms of the level of performance to be achieved on a measure or indicator. In these terms, if a statement does not refer to a measure it is not a standard.
- *Understandable*. Readily and easily understood by all, especially newcomers. This is more likely if staff take part in clarifying quality features and in formulating standards.
- *Behavioural*. Stated in terms that make clear what behaviour is required.
- *Grammatical*. With a subject, verb and object.
- *Achievable*. Too-high standards can be demoralizing.

Quality experts debate whether standards should be defined in terms of absolute ideals, minimum requirements or realistic levels. In the framework presented here, standards are levels of performance to be achieved on defined measures. Those who formulate the standards at the same time set the level to be achieved. They may use benchmark data (e.g. current best performance in the market) or absolute ideals (e.g. 100%, or zero error). These levels (the current standards) are always interim targets towards an absolute ideal.

Formulating standards — steps

There are several ways to formulate or set standards. The following describes the approach developed in the research to specify standards that meet the above criteria for a 'good' standard. These steps are technical and social — the latter concerning who is involved and how.

Formulating standards: 'technical' steps

The starting point is a general statement of a subject or area that is important (a quality feature). The result of the steps — the standard — is specified in terms of a level of performance to be achieved on an indicator or measure.

In the early stages of a quality programme:

1 Starting from the requirements and the flow-process chart, define the things it is important that the service should do — the quality features. Identify these in terms of the three dimensions of Client, Professional and Management Quality.

2 Prioritize: pick out the most important quality features at present — the things which, if the service did better, would do the most to improve quality.

3 Take each quality feature and focus on the essential aspect: look for things that would indicate whether the service was doing well or badly in relation to that subject. (This moves from a general abstract statement to a specific statement of something that can be observed or judged.)

4 Decide how performance will be measured and documented.

5 Specify the standard, in terms of a statement of the level of performance to be achieved on the measure or indicator.

With this standard established, the service can measure performance and judge the effects of any corrective actions.

These technical steps should be used to formulate Client, Professional and Management Quality standards. In our research, we found that in the early stages of a quality programme no more than the six most important quality features for each of the three dimensions of quality should be chosen to establish a set of 18.

Later a service will widen its list of quality features and choose more standards to measure at different intervals. It will define quality features from market research and from the work done on the business strategy and link the operational Quality Management Cycle to the strategy process.

Note that a collection of standards formulated in this way is not a quality system (see Chapter 7). A quality system is based on underlying theory about what needs to be done to provide a quality service (e.g. management responsibilities, training). It is possible to assess a service to check whether it is doing all of the things thought necessary to assure quality, but this is different from the service assessing its own performance in relation to market-defined quality features.

The box above shows the 'technical' steps of honing down

abstract statements to specific and observable events, so as to produce the right kind of statement. Just as important as these steps are the 'social' steps.

Formulating standards: social steps

1 Establish working groups to consider the service from the Client, Professional and Management Quality dimensions, and to clarify the quality features of the service.
2 Each group proposes a set of standards for the dimension they consider.
3 A combined working group brings together these sets to identify standards which overlap or duplicate, and which may be combined in one.
4 Identify conflicting as well as compatible standards.
5 Decide priority standards and rationale for this, or negotiate acceptable balances between conflicting standards.

The social steps are important for involving those who work in the service and will have to achieve the standards. These steps make it possible to recognize conflicts between standards and to work out priorities and ways of dealing with them — a 'political' rather than a technical process.

Formulating standards: common mistakes

1 Formulating standards for what is easy to specify, not what is important. Costly because of the time taken to set standards and measure something that is not of prime importance; the time then wasted trying to improve performance on the wrong things; and standards becoming discredited.
2 Formulating standards for everything early on in a quality programme.
3 Imposing on staff a detailed, ready worked-out set of standards, even if they are appropriate for the particular service.
  Often these mistakes are all made at the same time and staff begin to see quality as more pointless bureaucracy.

Incompatible standards

When the standards from different working groups are brought together (see box 'Formulating standards: social steps') there may be conflicting standards. That is, where the performance specified in one area would mean lower performance in another. Usually this arises from the need to meet the requirements of different interest groups. These conflicts will not be resolved in the realm of standard-writing, but in reality by working out accommodations and priorities with the interest groups themselves.

For example, one group of professionals decided that a priority problem was poor assessment, and defined assessment as a key quality feature. They identified the main cause as not enough time being spent on assessment. They formulated a standard, and a set of items that all assessments should cover. The group considering Client Quality decided that a priority problem was the length of waiting time for assessment. They set a standard of a minimum waiting time. When the sets were brought together it became clear that, given the staffing and the way the service was set up, it was not possible to meet both standards.

The decision was that the assessment standard was higher priority, but the debate clarified the reasons why. It enabled the group to devise ways of minimizing client dissatisfaction, to publicize and explain their waiting times, and to invite suggestions for improvements which would allow the assessment standard to be met.

Recognizing these conflicts is especially important to improving quality. Conflicts exist and continually undermine quality improvement unless they are addressed. Staff may not be aware of the conflicts, but they are there. For front-line staff, the energy taken up with wrestling with incompatible standards and having to keep deciding how the balance should be struck is a continual and unnecessary drain. Specification in this way brings the conflicts out in the open and makes it possible to recognize them and to work out ways of dealing with them, for example through negotiation.

One of the drawbacks of professional audit is that these conflicts are recognized too late. A full set of standards is not developed in a process like the one described above. Changes are proposed by professionals which conflict with other dimensions of quality, and this reinforces the professional–management divide. Worse, the opportunity to identify areas where quality can be improved on all dimensions is lost.

Using these technical and social steps, a full and balanced set of standards should be established for the service, made up of Client, Professional and Management Quality standards.

Before discussing the measurement part of the cycle we need to consider whether and how to specify the intangibles that are so important to Client Quality.

Specifying intangibles

Health services are not like manufacturing where you can specify physical outputs. But specification and measurement are essential to control and improve quality. Is it possible or necessary to specify that staff should care for clients, or be friendly or polite?

It is certainly important to understand and describe the behaviours thought to lead to client satisfaction. For training and guidance, staff need something more specific than 'just make sure he's happy'. But there are dangers in going too far and specifying these behaviours as standards and as part of a service's quality specification.

It may be appropriate in some services where the ends and means are known and prescribable and the client contact is short (e.g. McDonalds, supermarkets, Disneyland). In health services, the relationships are not just longer, but different. A client soon senses whether the people on whom they depend, often for their life, care about them and understand how they are feeling. This cannot be prescribed. There are also limits to the amount of specification appropriate for professionals if they are to be able to use discretion in assessing and treating clients.

Why then do some wish to specify the intangibles to this extent? Certainly specification and standard-setting are central to any quality approach, and 'intangibles' do account for a large part of the Client Quality of a service. However, the concern to specify 'intangibles' in health services may be a sign of the bureaucratic control culture approach to improvement, rather than an understanding of the quality approach.

Specification for measurement and control is different from being specific for training

In formulating standards and other specifications it is necessary to distinguish between the specifications to be used for measurement and control, and the things that need to be specified to give examples for guidance and training.

For training purposes it is necessary to be precise about what is expected of staff. For example specifying behaviours towards clients to show how to relax clients. However unlike with McDonalds, it is inappropriate to put all these specifications in a procedures manual and monitor what staff do against these specifications.

If the problem is getting staff to be caring, friendly and polite, there are better ways of doing this than specifying behaviours. Often staff ignore and resent over-specification of this type and it has the opposite effects to those intended. Sometimes it is the control culture that accounts for poor staff−client relationships, which are not improved by more control. They are improved by describing clearly the ideal behaviours and making changes to working environments and management relationships to help staff develop appropriate attitudes towards and relationships with clients. Set standards for outcome (e.g. client satisfaction), not for every interaction with the client.

Cost-effective standard-setting

● Select what it is important to specify (quality feature) and understand why it is important to specify it
● Use a technical method to hone down abstract and ambiguous statements into standard statements that cannot be misinterpreted, and are also clear enough for anyone to establish whether what is intended is happening
● Ensure that all the relevant people understand what is expected and why, not by giving them a clear standard statement but by involving them in formulating the statements.
● Recognize and address conflicting standards, and invest in areas where quality can be improved in all dimensions at the same time.

Cycle Part 3: Measurement

The next part of the Quality Management Cycle is comparing what is done with what was intended — measuring performance in relation to standards. Previous chapters considered methods for measuring Client, Professional and Management Quality performance. Here we consider general issues of measurement.

The purposes of measurement are:
● To decide if action is necessary
● For people to judge the effect of their efforts on the important things
● To allow exact communication

Measurement is a tool for helping people communicate with each other more effectively — to communicate a perception or observation in terms of 'how much'.

Monitoring and measurement

Monitoring — observing past or present activity in relation to a standard or an implicit or explicit criteria or

106

specification (e.g. did the nurse follow procedure?).

Although the two terms are used interchangeably, measurement is more sophisticated:

Measurement — the comparison of something with a fixed unit.

Monitoring is 'yes or no', measurement is 'how much'. Measurement makes comparison possible with similar things elsewhere, or through time.

Count measures are based on judging whether an event falls within a particular category (e.g. counting errors or complaints).

Rating measures are ways in which people can express their judgement of the amount of a specified something by rating the amount on a scale (e.g. 'on a scale of 1–10 I would rate the politeness of the receptionist as 6').

- What gets measured gets done
- If you can't measure it, it's not quality
- If something cannot be measured, it cannot be improved
- Measurement for someone else is often less accurate than measurement for your own purposes

Many newcomers to the quality approach recognize the importance of measurement, but make the mistake of starting there. The starting point is deciding what is important, then specification, and then deciding what methods to use to measure performance.

Everything can be measured. For example, if clients say that politeness is important to them, it is because they are affected by it and can make judgments about how polite staff are. All they need is a rating scale to help articulate their judgements. The only problem is that different clients will be judging different things, hence it is important to help them to be specific so that more reliable comparisons of their judgements can be made. What is not at issue is a client's or anyone's ability to make a subjective judgement about something that is important to them. With the right assistance people can easily express their judgements in a way which is useful to a service wishing to make improvements.

Many assume that measurement is only about objective measures such as waiting times, temperature, or number of appointments, and that a subjective preference rating is not a measure. It is curious how service providers often wish to use indirect or objective measures, even when it is cheaper and more valid to measure through client ratings.

In many areas it is not possible or cost-effective to develop objective measures, and more important to establish some form of quantification of the subject of concern. Too often the tools take over — because a measurement method exists it is used, but it is actually less useful for the purpose than a cruder, cheaper method that measures the right thing less accurately.

Measurement is not complete without a record of the measurement data. Indeed it is sometimes difficult to distinguish the method of measurement from the method of documentation or recording (e.g. is a checklist a method of measurement or a method of documenting observations?). Documentation is important for making comparisons and to judge the effects of certain changes, as well as to allow long-term review and quality audit.

As a service extends its set of standards, decisions will have to be made about which standards to measure and report on frequently, and which to measure and report less frequently, perhaps as part of an annual quality review.

We now turn to the final parts of the Quality Management Cycle: analysis and presentation, and action. The previous chapter considered methods used in the action part of the cycle for corrective action. This chapter considers a more sophisticated approach to correction using statistical process control techniques.

Cycle Part 4: Analysis and presentation of quality data

The next part of the cycle is analysing and presenting the measurement data. Even in the early stages of a quality programme, the way performance is presented and analysed is important for ensuring that the most important problem is selected for action. The previous chapter considered how to choose priority problems for corrective action.

Graphs and charts are quality methods for representing data and process variations. They help to identify problems at an early stage and to work out the causes of problems. They are essential to process control and quality assurance (Chapter 7) and are important for representing and analysing data because they are easier to understand and to take in than lists of numbers.

Graphs and charts are also more likely to be looked at and discussed by staff groups and can be posted somewhere central. They also help people to become familiar with the characteristics of a process and with how the process is behaving, rather than only focusing on numbers compared to targets.

- Post this information in common work areas
- Time spent drawing up presentations can be reduced by a data gathering method which records data in a way which highlights trends

Graphs are easy to use and can be converted into control charts. The most common is a histogram for representing measurement data. It shows the variation any process has within it and whether the process is behaving as one would expect. Scatter diagrams are used to find out if there is any connection between two variables and to indicate (not prove) possible cause and effect relationships (Walton 1986).

Control charts are an extremely important part of the quality approach. They are powerful methods for making improvements and embody a fundamental quality philosophy: that the aim is not to meet specifications and allow variations within specification, but rather to produce process consistency through continual improvement.

Control charts (or Shewhart charts) are methods for understanding to what extent processes are under control and to what extent they are being improved. Control charts are quality methods that would be used within the Quality Management Cycle in the later stages of a quality programme. Rather than explain these charts just as a method for representing data, the following discusses them within the context of statistical process control methodology. This is a sophisticated approach to quality control and correction.

Statistical process control

Significant improvements can be made by staff using the methods described above within a Quality Management Cycle. One of the most powerful methodologies, statistical process control, is best introduced after staff have become familiar with both the Quality Management Cycle and the Quality Correction Cycle and with simple methods.

Control charts are a method of statistical process control that can be introduced in the action phase of the cycle to identify and eliminate problems. In the longer term, statistical process control methods will be used in all parts of the Quality Management Cycle. That is, many quality features and the way they are specified are determined by statistical control process methodology, as are the measurement methods and the methods for presentation and analysis of data and action. To control quality effectively it is important to know the variations, not the average performance.

To give a simple explanation of this more sophisticated approach to quality management, we can illustrate how it could be applied in an outpatient department. Many departments select waiting for consultation as a priority area for quality specification and specify a standard of 'less than one hour'.

Often departments can improve other aspects of the service, but find it more difficult to reach the waiting time standard. If staff were to use statistical methods they would use these methods to choose the most cost-effective way of sampling. They would use both a histogram and a scatter diagram to represent all the sampled times.

A histogram shows a distribution of times on each side of the average, similar to a normal distribution curve. A normal distribution is the typical bell-shaped curve showing the variation in a large sample, for example for variation in heights or weights of a population. The fact that certain waiting times do not fall within the normal distribution would alert staff to a quality problem. In simple terms the reasons are as follows.

In a normal distribution, over 95% of the times fall within two standard deviations of the average, and over 99% within three standard deviations. This makes it possible to specify upper and lower control limits. These limits represent the area within which most times should occur. It is a statistical fact that a point (here one waiting time) occurring more than three standard deviations from the average (outside of a control limit) is so unlikely that it must be due to a special reason (a 'special cause' (Deming) or 'assignable cause' (Shewhart)). It would be the occurrence of certain waiting times outside the statistically-predicted random variations that would alert staff to a quality problem.

Before using these statistical methods, it is likely that staff would have taken a variety of steps to try to reduce the average waiting time. A statistical approach would lead them to concentrate their attention on the waiting times outside the control limits, and to look for the causes using the problem-solving techniques already described. Often the problems do not lie within the service process, but some do. Essentially it is a waste of time to look for the cause of a chance variation, but a variation identified in the way described is likely to be due to an assignable cause and alerts staff to the fact that the process is out of control.

Statistical process control

- The aim is to ensure that the process is under control, not to meet a minimum standard.
- Although the starting point is an externally prescribed standard (e.g. 1 hour), this aspect of service quality is later specified in terms of upper and lower control limits,

which are derived from the measurement data itself.
- The control chart focuses effort and attention on the key problem areas: time is not wasted on improvements which have a minor effect on waiting times.
- Solving the problems which cause times outside the control limit improves the service process, and the *average* waiting time is steadily and automatically reduced.

The quality philosophy behind this approach is discussed as part of quality assurance and accreditation in the next chapter. But consider for the moment, if you were a purchaser, what would give you the best evidence of the likely performance of a service in relation to waiting times:

(a) Evidence from the service that in the past, the waiting times of the service were generally averaging higher than the quality standard specified (1 hour);

(b) A set of process control charts showing the same average performance, but also the variations outside control limits.

Which would give you more confidence that a provider would not only meet the standard, but continually improve this feature of quality over the contracted period?

Summary

- The aim of quality management is continuous quality improvement
- Quality management is the responsibility of staff and management
- It is accomplished by using proven cost-effective quality methods within a Quality Management Cycle and a Quality Correction Cycle.

There is no point in introducing a sophisticated quality system into a service that does not have a clear management structure. The first step is to specify the basics of organization, and in particular, staff responsibilities.

When beginning quality management, a service starts with a few quality features related to known problems. The Quality Management Cycle is established by setting standards, measuring performance and taking action to remove the causes of the problems. When the most pressing problems are resolved, the service widens its range of standards and relates the Quality Management Cycle to market data and business strategy. A complete set of standards is formed covering Client, Professional and Management Quality.

Statistical methods can then be used for corrective action. This approach moves the aim of quality management away from conforming to standards to process control and continuous process improvement. The methods used should be suited to the understanding and experience of staff.

In health services, specification and measurement has been imposed rather than being used within a Quality Management Cycle framework. The methods have been used more to meet minimum requirements than as tools for continual quality improvement.

A CCREDITATION IS ONLY as good as the standards against which providers are assessed, and does not assure high quality health care. One reason is that most accreditation only requires providers to show that they have met a set of performance standards in the past. For accreditation to be an assurance of quality, it must require providers to show that they have an effective quality system.

Introduction

In the UK, quality appeared on many NHS agendas as a serious item for the first time in 1990. Providers wondered how to establish professional audit, and how to demonstrate the quality of their service to purchasers, and in some cases to referrers and clients as well. Purchasers wanted to specify quality in contracts, as well as price and quantity.

Some were sceptical as to whether the NHS reforms would improve services, but felt that the risks would be reduced if purchasers paid as much attention to quality as to price and quantity. However, given the many changes and deadlines it was not surprising that quality was viewed as another re-quirement imposed by the reforms. Few recognized that quality is not a purchaser requirement to be met, but a philosophy, a set of methods and an organizational revolution which is essential to the competitive position and survival of a service; that quality improves customer service, cuts costs, and raises productivity. Fewer still recognized that continuous quality improvement must be driven by the service provider, not the purchaser. Those that did recognize this, and were aware of the experiences of manufacturing and commercial services in this field, were daunted by the magnitude of the task of introducing a quality approach into a health service — the subject of the next chapter.

This chapter considers quality assurance and quality con-trol and elaborates on some of the principles underlying the quality approach. It also considers different approaches to accreditation. It proposes that for accreditation to give assurance of future performance, it should not just assess a service's past performance, but should also assess its quality system. This means developing our knowledge of which quality systems are most effective in different health services.

Quality assurance and control

In the past, quality control meant checking an item before it went out, and discarding it if it was not good enough. Quality

control is now a part of quality assurance, the latter aiming
to predict and prevent problems. Quality control refers to
the day-to-day and immediate actions which service providers
take to maintain quality through the Quality Management
and Correction Cycles described in the last two chapters.

Quality control

'The process through which we measure actual quality
performance, compare it with standard and act on the
difference.' *Juran and Gryna (1980)*

Quality assurance

'A management system designed to give the maximum
confidence that a given acceptable level of quality of
service is being achieved with a minimum of total
expenditure.' *British Standards Institute (1987)*

Quality system

'The organizational structure, responsibilities,
procedures, processes and resources for implementing
quality management.' *British Standards Institute (1987)*

Quality audit

A documentation and review of a service's quality
system to find out if Quality Correction Cycles and
Quality Management Cycles are working to good effect.

Quality assurance utilizes quality control and the methods
of the Quality Management Cycle to assure the quality of a
service. Professional audit is a quality assurance activity.
The principle of quality assurance is illustrated in the difference between life insurance and life assurance. With life
insurance you or your family get financial compensation
when things go wrong. In contrast, life assurance guarantees
that you will receive a financial sum at a particular date.
The aim of quality assurance is to make sure nothing can go
wrong, rather than finding out if something has gone wrong
and making corrections — it is proactive not reactive.

Quality assurance is all the activities undertaken to predict
and prevent poor quality. The main way in which an organization assures quality is through a quality system. A quality
system establishes Quality Correction and Quality Management Cycles, and ensures that these cycles are being carried

out and improvements are being made. A quality system includes the processes, such as the quality cycles, and the structure and other arrangements to ensure and show that the processes are performed, such as documentation and training.

The most well-known quality system in the UK is the British Standard 5750 (1987), and in the USA the Malcum Baldridge National Quality Award system (Øvretveit 1989). Both are based on the same principles and philosophy of an integrated, systematic and comprehensive approach to quality within an organization as the way to assure quality. An application of BS 5750 in health services is discussed later in this chapter.

The need for quality assurance

It is easier to explain some of the reasons why many organizations have introduced quality assurance by looking at institutional purchasers in the manufacturing sector. In the past these purchasers were satisfied to know that a provider had ways of checking products before they left the factory. They were impressed to see a pile of rejects at the end of the production line, which they were told were scrapped because they did not meet other purchasers' specifications.

In more recent times, no manufacturing company that did this would get a contract. Purchasers are aware that they pay for the rejects and that the cost of production using this approach to quality is high. In addition, many purchasers are using modern manufacturing techniques and processes such as Just-in-Time that demand guaranteed quality. Promising that the product will be to the purchaser's requirements, or that after-sales corrections will be done swiftly, or that compensation is guaranteed, is no longer enough.

Institutional purchasers of manufactured goods only sign a contract after a full audit of the supplier's quality assurance procedures. The supplier has to prove to the purchaser that they use a series of procedures to ensure quality right from the beginning, and that they have a comprehensive quality system.

This involves showing that there are procedures to ensure quality from the first moment the customer contacts them, through agreeing specification to design. Then the procedures follow from prototype production, setting up production, controlling incoming raw materials, training and motivating staff, to identifying faults at the earliest possible moment and eliminating the root cause. Sometimes purchasers want suppliers to show process control charts. If there is a need to check the product before it goes out, this is taken as a sign of poor quality assurance arrangements.

Not all purchasers assess a supplier's quality system them-selves. They will accept registration by the British Standards Institute as proving that the supplier has a working and effective quality system — the BSI 'accredits' the supplier's quality system.

Although much is said in health services about 'total quality management', true quality assurance has hardly begun for a number of reasons.

Quality assurance in health services

Although true quality assurance has hardly begun in health services, there are pressures for change.

1 *Poor quality is less obvious to clients, and routine simple outcome measures have not yet been developed.* We cannot visit a hospital and see a pile of patients that were 'rejected' because surgery was not up to the customer's specification. Even if we did, we would not be impressed to know that doctors and managers checked patients before they went home, and if there were signs that the procedures were not up to scratch, they held on to the patients to re-do the surgery, or simply scrapped the patient as an irretrievable reject. We want to be assured that everything possible is done to ensure that we get what we need from our first contact with the service to our last.

2 *Clients for health services have not had the expertise and power to assess and demand quality.* UK purchasing authorities have the power to demand quality, and their expertise to assess quality is developing. They require evidence of quality outcomes and of quality assurance arrangements in the services which they purchase on behalf of their population.

Both health service clients and purchasers are becoming more aware of, and concerned about, a service's quality assurance: not just that it reduces its errors and deals with complaints swiftly. They want a guarantee that all clients will always get the highest quality service.

Many purchasers have also done their homework and recognize that quality assurance reduces the cost of the service and that there is no quality cost tradeoff in an effective quality programme. They want providers to introduce quality assurance to make the service less expensive to buy.

*How can we be sure that the quality of this service
is acceptable, and will continue to be so if we contract it?*

Accreditation is one answer to the above purchaser's
question. To reduce their risks, purchasers can gravitate
towards trying to specify many inputs and processes in their
contract negotiations with providers, but purchasers are not
the experts in service delivery and do not have the capacity
to monitor such detailed specifications.

What would make life easier is to be able to turn to a
specification developed by experts for the type of service
they wish to contract. Better still is to have the experts
judge the service independently and declare whether or not
it meets these specifications. This is accreditation.

What is accreditation?

Accreditation is similar to licensing or registration, but is
usually voluntary. It is the recognition by an accrediting
agency that an individual or organization meets certain
criteria set by that agency. The term is used to describe
both the process used by the agency to make the
assessment, and the outcome of the assessment, where
the individual or organization is recognized by an
accreditation award to have met the criteria.

Accrediting people

In the case of individual practitioners, professional
associations set criteria and accredit the person. In most
cases the state then uses the association's certification as
its criterion for registration or licensing. Thus an
individual must pass certain exams and supervised
practice to be awarded a certificate by a professional
association (accreditation) and then be registered by the
state (state registration or licensing). In the UK, health
employers use accreditation to assure basic competence
to practise, and in many cases can only employ state-
registered professionals (Øvretveit 1988). In the USA,
medical practitioners must be relicensed every few years,
like airline pilots.

Accrediting services

For services in the UK there are advisory agencies, but
these do not have established standards for assessment
(e.g. HAS, MAS (Kogan *et al.* 1984)). There are inspection
agencies for aspects of health service organization

(environmental health, health and safety) and for some
private services, as well as statutory systems for
registration (e.g. nursing homes). There are also
accreditation bodies for education. However, in 1991
there was no nationally recognized set of comprehensive
standards for health care provision and no agency which
could assess a service against these standards and
accredit a service. One project is assessing the viability of
such a set (Brooks & Pitt 1990).

In the UK, accreditation is also seen as a solution to other
problems and concerns which the 1990 reforms brought to
the fore. Providers do not like having to meet all the different
requirements of different purchasers. Some think that
accreditation could reduce these differences, and give one
set of targets to aim for. Some provider managers think that
accreditation could strengthen their hand in discussions with
clinicians about variations in clinical care.

Consumer organizations, unlike the government, fear that
quality will fall in the new health market, especially for
some clients. They see accreditation as a way to protect
standards of health care. This fear is shared by many professionals, who also recognize that accreditation could maintain and advance the threat to their power.

The association of health authorities (NAHAT) is concerned about consistency of quality for all clients served by
one provider, and across an area and the UK as a whole. The
latter is also a concern of regions and the government,
although the government is not convinced that accreditation
is the solution. Neither are they convinced of the cost-
effectiveness of the variety of inspection and advisory bodies
for different services, as well as those for aspects of the same
service. They are unhappy about the duplication which often
occurs, especially with the new role of the audit commission.
Others see accreditation as a way to ensure that providers
establish quality systems, rather than simply trying to prove
that they meet certain performance targets or a set of national
standards.

However, accreditation is not the solution to all these
concerns and there are different types of accreditation, each
appropriate to different problems. Research shows that many
types of accreditation do not assure quality of care and may
increase costs. This is evident both from the history of
accreditation of organizations and of individual practitioners
(Øvretveit 1988). It will be argued that this is because health
accreditation has not always required providers to have a
quality system, or in the few cases where it has, the systems
required are not appropriate.

118

Accreditation of past performance or of a quality system?

This chapter is interested in accreditation as a means of assuring quality: a certification that a provider will deliver a quality service. There are two approaches: first, to establish a set of quality performance standards to be met, and to assess a service against this set. Second, to establish an agreed approach to quality, a quality system, and assess whether the service uses such a system. It is also possible to combine these two approaches.

A quality system ensures that standards are set and monitored, that action is taken and evaluated and the whole process is documented. It ensures that the organization has the structures, procedures and staff trained continually to improve quality and to carry out the Quality Management Cycle. We note that specification and standards are an essential part of a quality system, and that a quality system uses externally specified standards such as professional requirements and those of purchasers.

A service could perform well in relation to a set of performance standards chosen by experts to indicate the quality of the service in a number of areas. However, this would not show whether the service had an effective quality system; only that the service had performed well in relation to certain standards in the past. It would not assure that the service would meet these standards in the future. Neither would it show that the service was organized to improve quality continuously. A set of performance standards without a quality system does not assure quality for purchasers, nor enable providers to improve quality continuously.

Some go further and argue that the only quality systems which effectively assure quality and continuous improvement use statistical process control. Deming (1986) proposes that purchasers should look for statistical evidence of quality: 'you will note from the control charts far better than any inspection can tell you what the distribution of quality is and what it will be tomorrow'.

In order to decide whether accreditation is appropriate in the UK, and if so what type is best, we need to be clearer about what we aim to achieve by accreditation. Is accreditation in the UK to be in terms of the performance of a service in relation to a set of standards, or of a quality system, or of both?

It is generally thought that accreditation itself assures quality, regardless of whether accreditation requires providers to have an effective quality system. I argued above that it does not. I will develop these points in discussing different approaches to accreditation and the standards or guidelines used in each approach. Each approach has a different purpose.

British Standards Institute quality system

The British Standards Institute (BSI) provides quality accreditation by assessing whether an organization has established a quality system within the BS 5750 guidelines: they register an organization's quality system.

The BSI system (BS 5750 1987) lays down guidelines and criteria for a quality system, based on the principles of the quality 'loop' (similar to the Quality Management Cycle discussed in Chapter 6). Many manufacturing companies have met this BSI standard for a quality system, which is increasingly important for winning contracts, especially in the defence sector.

The BSI are flexible in their assessments, stressing that the guidelines must be adapted and appropriate to the size and sector of the industry. They are also rigorous and to apply and be assessed takes considerable time and energy, even if an organization already has a well-developed system. Small businesses (3 or 4 staff) have been registered and there is no reason in principle why a health provider could not apply for registration; indeed a few are preparing to do so.

Applying the BSI quality system in health services

The only reported application of the BSI guidelines for a quality system in health services was by Rooney (1988). She considered four services in two districts, focusing on outpatients at the Royal Shrewsbury Hospital.

Rooney interviewed staff and studied the different services to find out whether the following features which were essential to the BSI quality system were present: information transfer, traceability, feedback loops, documented records, standards (or expectations implicit and explicit), identification of non-conforming service and corrective action. Her conclusion was that many of the features were present or could be developed, but that they were not brought together in a formal quality system.

Although the services did not introduce a BSI-derived quality system, she argued for its feasibility, especially in purchasing, catering, pharmacy, maintenance, laboratories and medical engineering. She proposed a draft system for health services, based on BS5750, which defined criteria to be met in 20 areas:

1 Management responsibility
   (e.g. there is a quality policy, organization, etc.)
2 Quality system
3 Planning
4 Health service planning and monitoring control

 5 Document control
 6 Purchasing
 7 Quality control
 8 Inspection measuring and test equipment
 9 Instructions
10 Patients' medical records
11 Quality records
12 Patient care
13 Control of non-conforming services
14 Corrective action
15 Handling, storage, package and delivery
16 Patient discharge
17 Internal quality audits
18 Training
19 Servicing
20 Statistical techniques

To return to the issue raised earlier: would accreditation to BSI standard assure a quality service? There is no doubt that it would assure a service had a quality system, but, I will argue, the BSI system is not appropriate at this time for health services.

Whilst the principles of the BSI system are sound, the benefits of application and possible registration by a health service would not justify the costs at the early stages of a quality programme. Although I am not as critical of the system as a more experienced quality consultant (Hutchins 1990), the system could risk discrediting the quality approach with staff who were not used to the methods and disciplines. Considerable work is needed just to apply for registration. The documentation procedures would not be popular with staff who were unfamiliar with the approach — simpler methods should be used first.

There was criticism that the system is not suited to services, and BSI have responded to this criticism with a recent draft system for service industries (BSI 1990). The criteria for the US National Quality Award provide a better basis for developing a service quality system, and can help to prepare for BSI registration (Appendix 3 and Øvretveit 1989). This approach has criteria for assessing the following areas of a service:
1 Quality leadership
2 Information and analysis
3 Strategic quality planning
4 Human resource utilization and quality training
5 Quality assurance processes and cycles
6 Quality results (internal)
7 Customer satisfaction.

What then are the approaches to accreditation for health services, and do any include requirements to establish a quality system?

Health service accreditation

> **Accreditation — one definition**
>
> Quoted by Brookes, in her introduction to Sketris (1988): 'The professional and national recognition reserved for faculties that provide high quality health care. This means that the particular health care facility has voluntarily sought to be measured against high professional standards and is in substantial compliance with them.' (Lewis 1984).

This book argued that there is more to quality than high professional standards, which Lewis's definition of accreditation emphasizes. Brookes notes that common to all accreditation systems are an accreditation board, comprehensive standards continually updated to reflect current practice, and site visits by surveyors who assess the provider against standards and who make recommendations to the board.

From Sketris's (1988) study of accreditation in seven countries we can see similar structures and processes. Most accrediting organizations are private and the boards are dominated by medical membership from professional associations, with the exception of Spain. Their main source of income is from fees for an accreditation survey paid by providers. Although providers take part voluntarily, accreditation is usually a precondition for professional training, reduced insurance premiums, and for providers' receiving payment from national agencies for certain patients' care (although 'continued financial support from government' was viewed by one group as the least important benefit of accreditation (Duckett *et al.* 1980)).

A survey of a provider is usually undertaken by a team consisting of a doctor, a nurse, and an administrator, who are usually full time employees of the accrediting organization. They rate the provider's compliance against a set of standards, which is nationally debated and publicized. Few providers are refused accreditation (2% in the USA (Roberts *et al.* 1987)), not least because accrediting agencies fear being sued for the losses which a provider may suffer as a result of refusal.

Although there are similarities at a general level, different approaches to accreditation have been developed as the focus of concern has changed. The most marked differences are in the subjects for standards, and in particular, whether there are standards for a quality system and what these standards cover. This is most clearly illustrated in the history of accreditation in the USA, as in the fact that accreditation does not assure high quality health care.

Accreditation in the USA

In the USA there are two main systems: audit of individual patient care by contracted private review organizations, and organizational audit by a national accreditation agency used by the Medicare and Medicaid programmes (Joint Commission on Accreditation of Health Care Organizations).

In 1966 the federal government used three criteria to assure the quality of the services which they purchased for clients: accreditation by the Joint Commission, bed and service utilization reviews, and use of medical audit. By 1972 it was clear that these arrangements were not working to assure quality or hold costs down, and Professional Standards Review Organizations were established in regions to make sure utilization review and medical audit were effective. In the 1980s the system was changed, and Professional Review Organizations were contracted to check that aspects of quality were reviewed for the relevant patients.

Wilson (1989) argues that accreditation in the USA went through four phases, each with a different focus. We put to one side for a moment the objection that Wilson assumes that accreditation is the same thing as quality assurance, which it is only in a general sense. He describes how accreditation evolved in the USA as follows.

He describes the standards up to 1981 as being concerned with 'quality monitoring'. Here hospitals demonstrated quality by conducting medical and nursing audit on a percentage of admissions, patients or procedures. For two years after this, he describes the focus as being on evidence of action arising from the reviews, and that services used problem-solving cycles. He then describes attention shifting to a wider range of activities, with evidence required of 'comprehensive review' (the focus of Canadian accreditation). Finally he describes the current focus on standards of outcome. That is, actual results such as deaths, surgical complications, infection rates etc., and concurrent monitoring systems showing adverse patient occurrences (see the discussion of medical audit in Chapter 4).

Wilson's point about matching the accreditation approach and focus to the situation and expertise of providers is valid. It is relevant to the current debate on accreditation in the UK. For example, we do not have the knowledge and information systems to accredit according to outcome, and much debate surrounds the current outcome proposals in the USA.

However, I believe accreditation will only assure quality if standards require the key elements of a quality system (not just a quality programme or medical audit). We need to look at what it takes to assure quality in other industries, at modern theories of quality assurance, and develop a quality system that is appropriate to the UK health sector. From this, standards for accrediting quality systems in health can be developed, rather than using BSI or other generic systems.

Summary

- Quality assurance aims to predict and prevent problems, and to improve quality continuously, rather than inspecting output against standards after the event.
- Quality assurance aims to guarantee the quality of a service through quality control and quality methods.
- One way a provider can assure quality is to develop a quality system within their organization.
- Many view accreditation as the best way to assure health service quality. Accreditation at best is only as good as the standards against which providers are assessed.
- The experience of other countries shows that accreditation does not assure high quality health care.
- Often this is because accreditation does not require an effective quality system, or requires one that is not based on modern quality theories.
- Usually accreditation only requires the provider to show that they have met a set of performance standards in the past.

A FTER THE PRESENTATION *and discussion, the management team turned to the question of what they should do about quality. Some took the view that the approach was not really anything radically new — some simple techniques, and perhaps a variation of a management-by-objectives approach. What was needed was a training programme, some quality circles to solve the long-standing inter-departmental and inter-professional problems, and to work out what was needed to show purchasers that the service was doing something about quality.*

Debate turned to who would take the lead on quality, would there be a quality budget, and whether a quality specialist should be recruited. There were nods and murmurs of agreement to the view that there were pressing claims on the budget, and that other changes had to be carried out. The 'is it the right time/there's never a right time' argument began again.

There were some worried faces in the group. They were relieved that the practical members of the group were approaching the question in a business-like way, similar to the way in which they had approached the introduction of the new information system. Relieved, because at points they had become aware that a quality approach would mean a total revolution for the service, and they could not see how such a major change could be achieved at present. They were not sure that staff could or would change in the way implied — there did not seem to be any incentives. But on the other hand a half-hearted launch, with the lip service which was already becoming apparent, could discredit the approach, making it difficult to re-launch it properly at a later date. However, they went along with the suggestions because it seemed better to do something than nothing, and they could not suggest anything better.

Introduction

The point of this fable is to characterize two common re-actions to the quality approach, and the ideas about how to introduce quality which flow from these different under-standings. On the one hand, introducing a quality programme appears to be like any organizational change, but on the other hand it is nothing less than a complete transformation of how people think about and do their work.

There are two things that all quality experts agree on: that all staff must learn and use quality methods, and that top (and, I would add, middle) management must give leadership and be committed to quality. One survey of quality programmes found that the biggest single cause of failure was lack of understanding, commitment and leadership on the part of management.

Managers frequently fail to recognize the changes in working relationships and attitudes that are necessary, or are unable to change their role and relationships. Texts and introductions tend to stress the tools and methods, the 'engineering' side of quality. It is perhaps easier and less threatening to understand this aspect of the approach. However, throughout this book I have also emphasized human relations and the importance of changing organizational culture and people's attitudes towards work. Motivation and methods improve quality. I believe this to be the key to improving quality in public health services, given the values and professional background of many staff and the centrality of client–staff relationships. The starting point to making these changes is the way in which quality methods are introduced. If quality is imposed like many other changes have been in the past, it will fail, and traditional working relationships and attitudes will be reinforced.

It is because of my experience working with staff and managers introducing quality that the earlier chapters stressed the context in which the methods are used almost as much as the methods themselves. The aim must be to revive and release the creativity and energy that is there in the most apathetic and cynical, to enable staff to regain a sense of meaning and purpose in their work. A quality strategy serving a business strategy is a means to this end.

Quality plans and guidelines — terms

Quality strategy: a general and long-term plan (3–5 years) to change behaviour, culture and systems in a service to provide what clients require at the lowest cost, using quality methods and philosophies.
Quality programme: a shorter term plan (1–2 years) to achieve strategy objectives (e.g. establish quality costing and regular reports)
Quality project: a planned service improvement (often cross-departmental) with a specific aim to be achieved within 2 years, which contributes to the quality programme (e.g. meet defined quality standards for speed

and accuracy of transfer of information between hospital and GPs)

Quality policy: a general guide as to how an operational unit, a division, a unit, or a GP practice will carry out quality activities, and also the aims of these activities (e.g. type and frequency of surveys, complaints procedure, frequency of review of quality activities, arrangements for coordinating quality activities, prioritizing quality problems)

This chapter considers how to introduce a quality approach within a public health service. Although there is no simple standard formula and each service has to work out its own strategy, there are some basic principles which provide guidance, and the chapter outlines these. It concentrates on the two most important considerations in a quality strategy: phasing-in quality techniques, and changing culture and attitudes. It discusses the need to 'sell' quality to often indifferent or sceptical staff, and how to carry through the cultural changes which are necessary. It finishes by looking at different practical approaches to introducing quality.

Preconditions for introducing quality

The first precondition is to be clear about the boundaries of the unit involved. Is the aim to introduce quality within one ward, one department, a multidisciplinary team service, within a division made up of a number of these operational units, or across a unit as a whole? A manager will develop and introduce a quality strategy differently if they are part of an organization-wide quality drive to the way they will if they are 'going it alone', or with only 'lip-service' support.

Can managers go it alone? Is it possible to introduce a quality approach successfully in just one part of the organization? Some managers feel that because their organization has no quality policy or strategy they would get little real support and it would be too difficult to introduce a quality approach. Some see their main problems as being with suppliers and other departments. They have given up trying to change things because it causes trouble — how can you change the policies of the purchasing department or central supplies?

Isolation can make things more difficult, but it is no reason not to start doing something about quality — the 'brick walls' quickly turn into crumbling 'Berlin walls' when higher management is converted to quality. Much can be done within departments and services, and sooner or later a quality approach will be introduced — sooner if

127

individual departments show what they have achieved, and could achieve if their suppliers treated them as customers.

The second precondition is to be clear about responsibilities, in particular to clarify people's responsibilities for work processes by drafting flow-process diagrams (Chapter 3) and internal customer–supplier chains. Who is responsible for the performance of a service delivery unit and for the quality of that service? This question still lies unanswered in many units.

It is fashionable not to define responsibilities and to emphasize flexibility, and obviously over-detailed job descriptions are to be avoided. However, quality requires and forces clarity about responsibilities, both for the overall service and for sub-processes within the service — the 'ownership of processes.' A quality programme must start by clarifying responsibilities if they are unclear, otherwise there will be analysis but no action and improvement.

The third precondition is that there is business strategy which identifies the target clients and defines the quality features that are critical in the market. Chapter 2 argued that without this there is no context for a quality strategy and it is difficult to prioritize programmes and projects — there is no future in doing the same thing better if there is little demand or income.

Quality preconditions

● Be clear about the boundaries of the organization within which the quality approach is to be introduced
● Make sure responsibilities are clear, or use the early stages of the quality programme to clarify responsibilities
● Clarify the business strategy of the organization and the business aims which the quality strategy is to serve
● Gain the necessary quality competences. Do not give up because quality is not organization-wide. It soon will be, or it will be in your next job.

The end of this chapter looks at different approaches to introducing quality and at some practical steps. Before this, we consider what are, in my experience, the two most important ingredients of a successful strategy: phasing in quality techniques according to the capabilities and problems of the service, and developing the right culture and working relationships. It is important that the focus of different phases of the programme are compatible with staff expertise, appropriate to the market conditions, and that each phase builds on what has been established in an earlier phase. The following considers 'phasing quality' before turning to the second set of more complex subjects — cultural, attitudinal and relationship change.

Phasing-in and levels of quality sophistication

One of the most important principles derived from experience of introducing quality techniques is to introduce quality in phases. This is to maintain staff commitment and because this approach is more cost-effective: significant quality improvements can be made easily with simple methods early on.

> **The perils of quality over-saturation**
>
> Many managers and staff discount quality as another fad, but there are some whose enthusiasm exceeds their capacity to apply properly the changes. An example was a quality department, trained and converted to total quality, which joined forces with a service interested in 'doing something about quality' — or at least the manager was. The quality staff assigned sought out off-the-shelf quality specifications with lists of standards. Service staff were told that a quality service was one that met all the standards.
>
> Staff who were previously interested in and willing to use any good ideas which would help clients struggled to become familiar with the tome of standards and began to feel badly about how poorly they were doing. After trying to meet only a few they gave up in despair, their confidence shattered. Any further mention of quality was met with gloom, laughter or yawns. The manager and the quality experts concluded that it was difficult to get staff interested in quality and started looking at award schemes and motivation exercises.

A mistake second only to imposing a quality strategy without consultation with informed staff, is that of over-saturating the organization with quality techniques and demanding that they are all applied immediately, in particular, managers adopting wholesale, detailed specifications developed elsewhere at an early stage of a quality programme. This is frequently seen as a quick way of assuring others of the quality of the service, but it only ensures staff antagonism. The service is often not able to measure performance in relation to these specifications.

The earlier chapters proposed a selective approach: select a quality problem and start to use quality methods to resolve it in a Quality Correction Cycle (Chapter 5). Then select the key quality features and start a Quality Management Cycle (Chapter 6).

The following describes four phases for improving the quality of a service. Simple quality techniques are introduced first, which are easy for staff to use and produce tangible benefits for them and for clients. As the gains from a phase dwindles staff are then ready to use more sophisticated techniques which build on the specifications and models of the earlier phases.

Phasing quality

Start where the biggest improvements can be made for a low cost, and to go at a pace which staff can cope with.

Phase 1: clarifying objectives and responsibilities (getting organized)

Ensure that the foundations of organization are established before using quality methods.

Phase 2: overcoming outstanding quality problems (making fewer mistakes)

Not just by trying harder, but by using methods to find out and remove the root causes of problems in a systematic way through a Quality Correction Cycle.

Phase 3: developing quality management (covering all areas in a systematic way)

Establish the Quality Management Cycle and build a comprehensive set of standards and measure and control performance.

Phase 4: preventing quality problems by assurance (process control and controlling critical variables)

Use statistical process control methodology to control critical variables.

The aims are to keep staff interested, develop capabilities and systems systematically, and maximize return on investment. Each phase uses a set of techniques and involves a qualitative jump into a higher level of quality sophistication. Each phase uses different methods for specification and measurement (Chapter 6).

*Phase 1: clarifying objectives and responsibilities (getting
organized)*

The first phase is more about ensuring that the foundations of organization are established than about using special quality techniques. It is surprising how many services introduce quality approaches which flounder or are less effective because the basic organization structure and processes are so poor. Adding another layer of quality structures and processes over a complex or confused structure usually only adds further confusion and costs.

The aim of this phase is for staff to agree and understand the objectives of the service and responsibilities within it. Later stages of this phase involve clarifying responsibilities for sub-processes by drafting process-flow diagrams (Chapter 3).

*Phase 2: overcoming outstanding quality problems (making
fewer mistakes)*

The next phase is appropriate when staff are ready to make use of quality methods. That is, when they have learned how to use these methods and believe they need to apply them. It is about making fewer mistakes, not just by trying harder, but by using quality methods to find out and remove the root causes of problems in a systematic way.

The focus is on overcoming the most outstanding quality problems once and for all. This is the first step away from fire-fighting. In this phase, the service process is analysed to highlight and prioritize the key quality problems. Using a Quality Correction Cycle, each problem is analysed, causes identified and removed and the actions evaluated until the problem is overcome once and for all (see Chapter 5).

*Phase 3: developing quality management (covering all
areas in a systematic way)*

In maturing markets, success often lies in simply making fewer mistakes than competitors, and in health services phase 2 is likely to be appropriate for some time. But the need for continual improvement will require the service to move into a third phase which involves establishing a Quality Management Cycle and a comprehensive and balanced set of standards.

In time, staff become familiar with viewing their service and their own jobs as processes, and with the quality methods and systematic approach. As the most outstanding problems are eliminated using these methods, the service establishes a full set of Client, Professional and Management Quality standards. Staff develop measures and methods of documenting and presenting performance. They also develop their ability to select priority problems and to work on them using the problem-solving methods learned in the last phase, and start to make use of statistical methods to resolve problems.

Phase 4: preventing quality problems by assurance (process control and controlling critical variables)

This is a more sophisticated phase which fully moves into prevention. In this phase, specification focuses on the things which vary and which, if they are not controlled within a certain range, will threaten quality. All service inputs and processes are analysed to identify the critical variables and control charts are devised and refined to assure quality. In this phase the service can begin Total Quality Management.

The general principles of phasing are to start where the biggest improvements can be made for a low cost, and to go at a pace which people can cope with. It is a waste of money to build a detailed quality system if responsibilities are not clear and if people cannot understand the system or give the time to work it. Detailed systems and sophisticated techniques come later when people are ready for them, when the foundations are there to support the system and when the early easy gains have been made.

One of the problems faced by provider units is that purchasing authorities have begun to prescribe how quality should be introduced. In particular they have required providers to produce and adopt a set of quality standards. To some extent this is appropriate and necessary, especially in relation to outcome standards, but purchasers sometimes cross the boundary and prescribe in too much detail. They should be concerned about the progress the provider is making in establishing a quality system, and with assessing this system, rather than with the detailed standards.

We can now turn to a second set of issues concerning how quality is presented to staff to gain their commitment, and how to change culture and working relationships.

Creating a quality service culture

Half of quality is giving people effective tools to identify and to get to grips with the key problems. Training people to use these tools is easy. But training is a waste of money if people cannot or do not want to use the methods. The other half of quality is establishing a quality philosophy throughout the service and a culture that values quality. To do this it is usually necessary to change organizational structure and relationships, but also to take action consciously to change the culture of the service.

'Off-the-shelf' quality programmes can be force-fitted into a service — some developed for manufacturing are used in commercial and now public services. The argument is: change behaviour and changes to attitudes and culture will follow. Some of these programmes are successful for a short time. But unless the programme directly addresses health service culture or happens to be suited to the culture, it dwindles rather than gathering momentum and producing the continual quality improvements that are the aim.

'Culture' tends to be a catch-all term used to explain something which people find difficult to explain ('history' is another). Structural changes, such as changing and defining roles and relationships and developing teamwork help to change culture. Leadership by example is also important.

However, the approach taken here focuses on attitudes. The assumptions are that (i) attitudes are the key to changing culture, and (ii) attitudes to quality are best changed by showing staff that there are tangible benefits for them in improving quality, and that quality is a way of upholding professional and caring values.

What is organizational culture?

• The culture of service is made up of the behaviours, actions, language, customs and attitudes that are taken for granted
• Culture constructs and controls how people perceive the world and how they act, but it does so without people being aware of its influence. People produce and reproduce the culture in their everyday acts.
• The culture is related to the values that people hold and it gives sense and meaning to working life.
   Culture is revealed
• In formal and informal status hierarchies
• By looking at the actions and the people that are formally and informally valued in the service (e.g. a respected secretary, manager, or practitioner).
• In the language (e.g. the non-professional words commonly used to categorize clients, or to describe 'difficult' or 'good' clients, or a successful worker).
• In images and myths — the often retold stories about the last manager, or what one of the staff once did.

To change culture and to introduce a quality philosophy the starting point is to understand and respond to different staff attitudes. We need to know how different staff groups perceive and are likely to respond to a quality programme.

Staff attitudes towards quality

'It's another management con to get us to work harder. What's in it for us?'

'We're expected to do all these new things and to put the customer first, but they don't give us time or training — we do it on top of what we always did. With all this work you can't help resenting customers after a while.'

'It will pass when the general manager moves on. Just humour them and keep them out of our way — we've got a job to do'

Often we think we know or could guess how different staff perceive quality. Because so much is at stake it is important to find out for sure, either by surveys or group meetings and discussions, before launching a quality strategy.

It is useful to clarify three different sets of attitudes:
1 Attitudes which either make it difficult for staff to hear what is being said about quality (e.g. blockages due to fear), or which result in a passive resistance to quality;
2 Attitudes which result in an active resistance or opposition to quality, and,
3 Attitudes that could potentially support quality changes.

Once different staff groups are identified in terms of their attitudes, and the nature and causes of these attitudes are understood, it is possible to plan how to respond to and alter these perceptions (see box below). Understanding staff perceptions towards quality helps to decide how to present quality to different staff groups in a way which responds to their indifference or objections.

Internal marketing of quality

Understanding and responding to staff attitudes is part of internal marketing of quality. There is a need to 'sell' service quality to staff before trying to convince external customers. You cannot convince outsiders of the quality of a service if staff do not believe in it, and staff are often the severest critics.

Internal marketing involves understanding what different staff want from their work, designing quality programmes to

Understanding and responding to staff attitudes — a precondition for changing culture

	Attitudes towards quality	Responses in strategy
	Passive resistance	*How to reduce*
Staff Professionals Management	e.g. Fears, anxieties; Suspicion, scepticism; Revealed to be inadequate	e.g. Information, no job losses; Spell out what it means
	Active resistance	*How to neutralize/ transform*
Staff Professionals Management	e.g. Objections; Perceived disincentives; What stand to lose e.g. power or status; More work	e.g. Staff involvement; Recognition of quality change
	Potential support	*How to realize and nurture*
Staff Professionals Management	e.g. Could make work less frustrating; Job security in competitive markets; Acquire quality skill good for career	e.g. Reinforce positives; Give support to those interested

meet their needs and presenting quality in a way that shows how it meets their needs.

The idea behind the concept of internal marketing extends further than 'selling' a quality strategy. It also describes employers' approaches to shaping jobs to employees needs, in part because of competitive labour markets. The concept recognizes that all staff are in an exchange relationship with their employers, and that their employers must provide for staff needs if they are to attract and retain staff.

It is difficult for staff to care for clients if they are not cared for by their employers. (My experience in some hospitals suggests that the converse is not true — when staff are treated well it does not always follow that they treat clients well.) Generally there are parallels in the relationships between management and staff, and between staff and clients. And clearly staff wish to work in a service with a quality culture. A quality culture is important not just to compete for clients but to compete in a labour market for increasingly scarce health service staff.

Finding out about staff attitudes is not just in order to decide how to present quality. Their views really must be considered and real changes made in response. Understanding and responding to staff attitudes itself begins to change culture. Likewise if there is no real response to staff concerns, the exercise may well entrench attitudes.

As a result of attitude analyses and working to change culture, I have formed a view of the concerns of staff and of how quality is best presented and pursued. One of my starting points was the curious phenomenon that talk about improving health service quality was met with derision and suspicion. How is this possible? The following develops the argument that the best way to present quality is to show how it advances staff values, as well as providing tangible benefits.

Values and motivation

Morale is low in many services where staff have been worn down by years of under-staffing and continual cuts. There is cynicism about management pronouncements and promises, and government reforms, and concern about the direction in which the current changes may take the service. Those who do not fear for their jobs in the new 'market' environment worry that decisions will be made purely on cost criteria, and that savings will not go into better services.

For many the commercial and financial language and thinking that goes with the changes is unsettling. It undermines the professional ethos and, in public health services, the values of equal access for all and provision according to need. A chain of demoralization has set in in many services — a downward spiral of poor quality (Fig. 8.1). (This vicious circle is the opposite of the circle of quality improvement described in Chapter 5.)

The main way to change a service culture is to inspire staff with an idea that is consistent with the values they hold, and which helps them to make meaningful changes. A quality service culture is instilled when staff find that quality not only fits with their values and helps to crystallize their

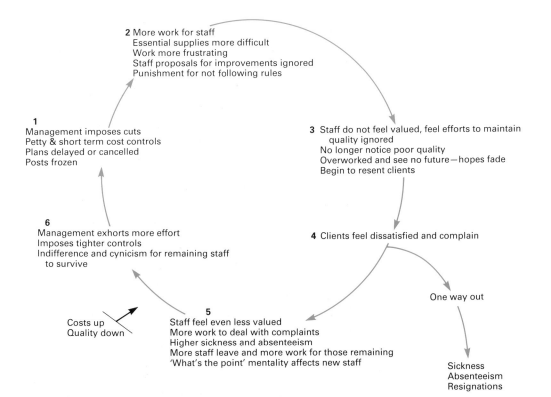

Fig. 8.1 The effects of poor quality.

desires for the future, but when they find that it also works — that it does enable them to bring about meaningful change.

This provides a clue as to how to introduce quality and change culture: demonstrate to staff how the quality approach links with their values and motivations. It also alerts us to one barrier to cultural change in the British and other public health services: that quality is perceived as another demand imposed by senior management and by a government which many see as holding values and aims opposed to a public health service. For some, quality is another Trojan horse in the long war of NHS attrition and must be bad simply because government and senior management wish to introduce it.

Quality is, and can be presented as, a way in which staff can uphold professional and service standards. Cynicism after all is often the only socially acceptable way of expressing despair. Quality provides staff with a weapon against the decline, and a way of ensuring that clients do not suffer from the reforms. It gives staff a way of testing what management are saying about changes being made to improve patient care, and gives them control over some changes.

137

Tangible benefits — what is in it for us?

However, the motive to defend and improve services to clients is not sufficient to power a quality strategy. Reason and argument rarely convince cynics or kindle the fire of action. For a strategy to work there has to be something tangible in it for staff and managers. The strategy has to be presented to make these benefits clear — it has to be 'sold' to staff.

Research into motivation and job satisfaction gives some ideas about the tangible benefits of quality for staff. Most staff do not work in health services just for the money. Although in some areas health is the only employer, there are usually jobs with better pay and conditions. In any job there are intrinsic satisfactions and a sense of achievement and pride that comes from doing the job well. This is as true for the worst kitchen, laundry and sluice maintenance jobs as it is for management accounting, district nursing and surgery. The intrinsic satisfactions of the job motivate people to do better, or at least to come back to work the next day.

> **Show how quality upholds staff values *and* provides tangible benefits**
>
> The most valuable things in the service are the professionalism and commitment of staff, which have been eroded and need to be nurtured. Quality reverses the downward spiral. A quality approach can be introduced in a way that connects with staff values and concerns and offers a realistic and worthwhile way forward.
>
> However, quality should not be presented only as a way of defending a service, or as something which resonates with and advances core values. It also has to be shown to provide something tangible for staff, as something that will help them protect their jobs and acquire necessary skills in competitive markets and as something which will save time in the long run, and remove the headaches and common complaints at work.

If introduced in the right way, a quality approach taps into this pride and motivation. It makes it possible for people to keep improving their service and to show that they are doing so. Quality should be presented in a way that shows staff how it will make their work more intrinsically satisfying. This can be done by showing how staff can use quality methods to overcome the headaches and time-wasting that stands between them and a good job, and that can make working life such a chore.

Just as important is the satisfaction of helping a client, and the client's recognition of a staff member's proficiency. It is a proficiency made possible because of the quality of the service process and organization. A major source of job dissatisfaction is being criticized by clients for poor treatment that a staff member knows was poor, but which they could not have given any better because of the system, the rules and other people's indifference.

When the same problem and complaint keep happening, staff tend to ignore it to keep their self-respect. Staff know that clients think they are less competent, when in fact they are handicapped by ineffectual systems and poor environments. Quality needs to be presented to staff so that they can see how quality techniques and attitudes will increase client satisfaction, which in turn will make their work more enjoyable.

Besides recognition and valuation by clients, a further motivator is recognition by superiors and peers. All too often staff spend time improving the service and their effort or the results are not recognized, or their conscientiousness is exploited. A quality approach first ensures that time and effort is spent on the right things and gets results, and secondly it makes the effort visible through specification and measurement.

Colleagues' and managers' recognition and valuation of a person's achievements are too rare in health services. It is important that a strategy provides ways of formally and informally recognizing and rewarding achievements. Management literature describes many proven ways of doing this, although quality experts disagree about individual or team pay incentives. It is also important to present quality to staff as something that will help them do more with less effort, and which will make good and poor performances visible, but in a way which is not threatening.

Quality: what is in it for staff?

• A way in which staff can uphold professional and service standards
• Increases intrinsic satisfaction of work and the sense of achievement and pride that comes from doing the job well
• Makes it possible for people to make continual improvements and to measure their progress
• Overcomes the headaches and time-wasting that

stands between them and a good job, and that can make working life such a chore
• The satisfaction of helping a client, and the client's recognition of a staff member's proficiency
• Fewer dissatisfied and irate clients
• Makes the effort visible through specification and measurement
• Colleagues' and managers' recognition and valuation of a person's achievements
• Ensures that time and effort is spent on the right things and gets results — can do more with less effort
• New quality skills and experience are increasingly necessary in the job market

These then are some ways in which quality can be presented to staff to make it an integral part of the service. A strategy should:
• Aim to change the service culture by appealing to staff values and motivations
• Build on professional values and be introduced with an understanding of staff attitudes towards quality
• Show how quality helps staff to overcome the problems that make their work less satisfying, and that quality improvements will be recognized and rewarded
• Provide, and be seen to provide, a way for staff to do something about their concerns and take control of their situation

Quality strategies

In practical terms, how then should a manager introduce a quality approach into his or her service, be it a ward, team, division or unit? One way is an organization-wide project-based approach, another a departmental or unit quality system development approach.

The first approach is 'top-down' and starts with top and middle management quality awareness and commitment. A top-level quality council is formed, which commissions an audit of the quality status of the service (see Appendices 2 or 3) and identifies or prioritizes quality problems. They establish project teams (usually interdepartmental or inter-disciplinary) to address the key problems and to learn and apply quality tools and techniques to solve these problems.

This approach may get the highest return investment in the early stages, but it risks not introducing quality into all areas of the service, and not developing quality systems essential to long-term continual improvement.

The second approach is 'bottom-up' and focuses on operational units developing their own quality system. An example is a department specifying and improving service in successive phases, such as those described in the first section of this chapter. The advantage of this approach is a steady improvement to quality through developing a quality system. Disadvantages are potentially missing interdepartmental problems, and uneven or ineffective quality initiatives. In practice, a mixture of both approaches can be used.

Rather than following the quality experts' steps in detail, the best way is for a service to decide its own approach drawing on:
• Experts' steps, and their assumptions and principles
• Research into why quality programmes fail and what works under which conditions
• An understanding of what you will mean by quality
• An understanding of the service history — in the past what changes worked/did not and why?
But have a Plan and review it.

Considerations in formulating a quality strategy

Aim for

• *Train all staff* to use simple quality methods, to identify priority problems, to get evidence of causes, to remedy causes and evaluate effects
• *Use methods*: make sure staff use these methods and that successes are recognized
• *Phased building*: introduce simple quality methods and establish the value of the approach before using more sophisticated techniques
• *Higher management follow-through*: assess managers in terms of whether they make changes in response to problems staff cannot resolve themselves (e.g. suppliers)

Consider

• *Staff attitudes towards quality*: identify fears, resistances and assisting forces, and formulate a strategy to respond to and change perceptions about quality.
• *Service culture*: use knowledge of attitudes towards quality to understand the culture of the service. Develop the strategy in relation to the values, attitudes and motives of staff — what they are and what they need to be.
• *Learn lessons from previous changes*: understand what accounted for the success and failure of other changes in

the service, and carry out a strategy in the light of these lessons.

● *Participation*: ensure staff take part in formulating the quality plan, as well as in implementing and reviewing it.

● *Politics*: identify the interest groups in the service and consider what they have to gain and lose from a quality programme. What are the incentives and disincentives for a change of this type?

● *Audit the present quality status of the service*: assess the service using a quality audit (for example the one reproduced in Appendix 2, or the Maps-Qual system described in Appendix 3).

● *Decide which quality approach to use*: formulate the strategy to introduce and develop a quality approach which helps the service take a systematic and coordinated approach.

● *Management commitment*: the time and attention spent by managers on quality will signal its true importance. How management responds to quality initiatives from the grass roots can make or break a strategy.

Where management commitment is meagre, and investment resources even less, it is important not to launch an organization-wide quality strategy with a fanfare. It is an insult to staff to spend money promoting quality, leaving none left to make changes which staff know are essential. One approach is to concentrate resources on a pilot quality programme within one service delivery unit, the aim being to show what can be done, to build up experience, and to convert sceptical natives into ambassadors for the approach.

Example: a unit-wide approach to quality

● A quality group (different depts/professions/levels) with an understanding of quality proposes a programme to the Unit Management Board, as well as a suggested framework, guidance and a quality policy

● UMB decides programme and timetable (compatible with business plan)

● Sets expectations and targets for each service, e.g.

  ● to have identified the first priority quality improvement project, by...date

  ● to have a set of quality standards, formulated using X approach, by...date

- to have plans for cost-effective methods to get feedback from clients and referrers, by...date
- to have an estimate of the current costs of poor quality, by...date
- UMB to call for regular report of each service's progress on above
- Quality group to identify priority cross-departmental problems, propose project groups and oversee their progress
- Establish specialist quality support to advise line managers
- Training programme on quality methods and concepts for all
- Quality made part of service and individual's performance reviews
- Establish other ways of recognizing quality efforts
- UMB carry out regular reviews of programme and sustain momentum

Summary

1 *People and perfect processes make a quality service.* Other chapters concentrated on perfecting the processes using quality tools, but to introduce quality, the emphasis should be on the people part of the equation, and on creating a quality culture. Motivation is important as well as methods.

2 *Managers have responsibilities to their staff,* besides their responsibilities to clients and higher management. Putting the client first sometimes appears to conflict with staff welfare. It can mean disrupted breaks, long hours after work, and high pressure at peak periods, even in a well-organized service.

A high quality service is not one that meets clients needs and higher management requirements at the expense of staff welfare. Staff cannot devote their attention to meeting client needs if their own are not met and if they are overworked and exploited to reduce costs. Staff will rightly focus on self-protection and there will be no inner incentive to improving quality.

3 *Managers have to build a quality culture,* where staff gain satisfaction from meeting client needs and from continually improving quality. There is no contradiction in the quality approach between meeting the needs of clients and of staff — quality is a means of meeting both. The role of management in ensuring quality is central — in managing

workload, in ensuring that staff know what is expected and are given the means to do it, and in releasing the potential of staff to give good service to clients and gain satisfaction from doing so.

4 *A well-formulated and conducted quality strategy releases unsuspected energy and creativity within the organization.* The cost of poor quality was noted earlier, but the greatest cost cannot be quantified — this is the cost to the organization of the corrosive effect on employees of accepting poor quality — 'Let it go, no-one will notice.' After a time, even staff do not notice. Those who do leave, increasing recruitment and induction costs. It may not be a free market for clients, but it is for staff, and it is a seller's market.

5 *Poor quality de-motivates,* makes people think it is not worth the effort to get things right, and becomes ignored or accepted as part of working life. It produces a chain of demoralization. The most important quality source is each person's inner desire to do a good job, and to please customers and management. The most important incentive is inner satisfaction and pride from doing a good job, and recognition from clients and management. This comes from assuming responsibility for quality, and from making quality improvements successfully because one has the training and support to do so.

6 *Most organizations only have one chance to play the quality card.* If they get it wrong, staff and clients will not believe a re-launch or re-introduction — quality becomes discredited (this has already happened with quality circles in some companies). Meanwhile, the competition might have got it right and it will be too late to catch up. With so much at stake it is important to plan and manage the introduction of quality with care.

The biggest asset is that significant improvements can be made easily early on. Proving the value of the approach is the best way to get take-up. The gains are not just the calculable cost savings, but the removal of long-standing frustrations — the effect of this on staff may be more valuable.

A *SYSTEMATIC APPROACH, understood and applied by all staff, is the key to continuous quality improvement. The 'Wel-Qual Framework' is one approach developed for health services. It links everyday quality management to overall business strategy. This ensures that improvements are made that are critical to the service's future market performance.*

Introduction

This chapter presents a framework for developing a service strategy and a quality system, termed the 'Wel-Qual Framework'. The framework provides guidelines for developing a comprehensive approach to quality. It also serves as a summary of the book and shows the links between the subjects considered in earlier chapters.

The principles apply to an operational unit or sub-service within a larger unit (e.g. a surgical directorate, a support service), or to a general practice. The framework shows which elements of the business environment to consider in formulating the sub-service strategy. A service carries out research to find out what the business environment requires of it, and defines these external requirements in a 'service brief'. Staff working at the operational level use this data as the basis for their quality management. In this part of the framework, staff use the market research and other data to select the quality features which are the start of the Quality Management Cycle.

The framework shows the steps and necessary links from market research and strategy to operational quality management. The structure and process for doing the work of each stage and ensuring the links is a separate issue. Most services are changing their structures to respond to the health market (Chapter 2). The emphasis in this chapter is on making sure staff at the operational level know what is important to success in the market, and use this information in their quality management.

The 'Wel-Qual framework'

The framework (Fig. 9.1) links business strategy (Parts 1–4) to the Quality Management Cycle (Parts 5 and 6) to ensure that quality improvements are related to the business environment. It covers the initial work of mapping the business environment (Part 1) and then defining what is required of the service if it is to compete successfully in future markets (Part 2). (More details of what is involved in these first parts

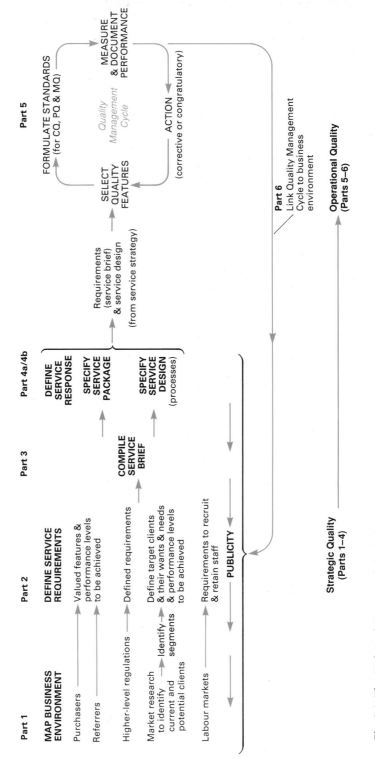

Fig. 9.1 The Wel-Qual Framework for linking operational quality to business environment.

of the framework are to be found in the discussion of service strategy in Chapter 2. The framework concentrates first on the 'needs' part of the service success equation, and then turns to the 'response' part of the equation in Parts 3 and 4 below.)

The framework then shows how the different external requirements of the service are converted into a definition of the 'service package', and into specifications of what the service has to do to meet the requirements (Parts 3, 4a and 4b). These internal specifications then form the basis for service operation and the Quality Management Cycle (Part 5 of the framework) that was discussed in Chapter 6. Part 6 of the framework shows that the Quality Management Cycle must be related to the business strategy in regular reviews.

Part 1: mapping the business environment

The first part of the framework divides the business environment into purchasers, referrers, higher-level regulations, clients, and staff labour markets (Fig. 9.2). It involves clarifying who are the potential purchasers for the service (public authorities and others), the potential referrers, and the higher-level requirements of the service which predefine what can be done and how (e.g. national, regional or district policies and directives, and other legal, environmental, health and safety regulations).

To contribute to this 'broad-brush' mapping, a service conducts local market research to identify who are the potential future clients for the general type of service contemplated at this stage. Discussions and negotiations are held with potential purchasers and referrers to find out who they see to be the future clientele for the service.

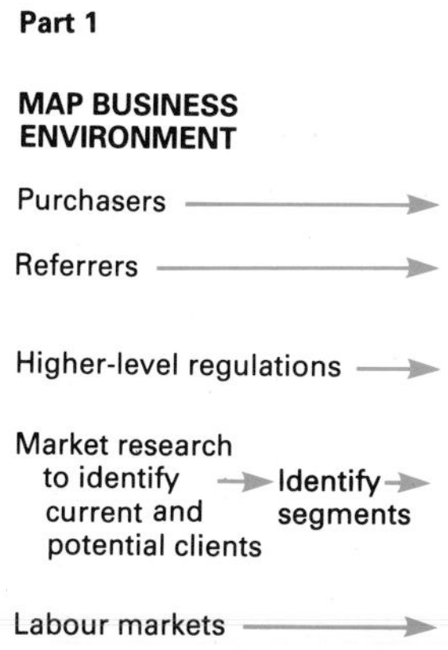

Part 1

**MAP BUSINESS
ENVIRONMENT**

Purchasers ⟶

Referrers ⟶

Higher-level regulations ⟶

Market research
  to identify ⟶ Identify ⟶
  current and   segments
  potential clients

Labour markets ⟶

Fig. 9.2 Part 1: Mapping the business environment.

The market also involves a labour market and other potential providers. Information is gathered about the future labour market for the different staff groups who will provide the service. Information is also needed about potential competitors and their current performance, which is regularly updated. To complete the mapping of the business environment, a profile of the current service is compiled, defining what services are provided to whom at what cost.

Part 2: defining requirements

Part 1 identifies the key parts of the business environment. In Part 2 (Fig. 9.3), the service takes each element of the business environment and defines what is required of the service if it is to compete successfully in future markets. This involves finding out what purchasers and referrers want the service to provide, and how they rate the current performance of the service on these features in comparison to the alternatives. Purchasers and referrers are asked to define the key features of service and what level of performance they want.

Part 1	**Part 2**	**Part 3**
MAP BUSINESS ENVIRONMENT	**DEFINE SERVICE REQUIREMENTS**	
Purchasers ⟶	Valued features & performance levels	
Referrers ⟶	to be achieved	
Higher-level regulations ⟶	Defined requirements	**COMPILE SERVICE BRIEF** ⟶
Market research to identify ⟶ Identify ⟶ current and segments potential clients	Define target clients & their wants & needs & performance levels to be achieved	
Labour markets ⟶	Requirements to recruit & retain staff	

Fig. 9.3 Part 2: Defining requirements.

It also involves defining the target clients segments revealed in the market research (see Chapter 2 for the detailed steps). Further market research is then done with the target client groups to establish their valued features of service, and what level of performance they want on each of these features (see Chapter 3).

Work is also done with professional service providers and referrers to define what they judge client needs to be, and the level of performance to be attained to meet these professionally assessed needs. This completes the 'needs' part of the equation described in Chapter 2.

Last but not least are the requirements for recruiting,

retaining and developing the different staff groups who are likely to be needed to provide a high quality service (e.g. clarifying pay, conditions, professional training and other needs). In Part 3 of the framework below, these staff requirements are converted into specifications of what the service must do to attract and retain staff, and how much it will cost.

These first parts of the framework give a detailed list of the different requirements from the point of view of the key interest groups. The requirements are defined in a way which makes it possible to judge how well a service is meeting these requirements. The next parts are concerned with converting these external requirements into specifications of how the service should respond and operate if it is to meet these requirements.

Part 3: service brief

Because the different requirements are specified, the overlapping or conflicting requirements become clear at a relatively early stage. For example purchasers may want a certain service capacity at a certain price. Referrers may want a higher capacity and fast response, as do clients and carers. It may be difficult to recruit certain staff groups.

These conflicts have to be addressed before it is possible to compile the final service brief. Although this is easier said than done, there is no point in designing a service or pursuing a service strategy which is riddled with contradictions. Too often management abdicate their responsibility for recognizing and addressing these conflicts, which then plague the operation of the service and are dealt with by front-line staff in different, often sub-optimal, ways.

There will always be tensions and conflict between the different requirements of the service, but the aim at this stage is to decide the best balance and trade-offs, and to be clear about the priorities. To minimize the tensions, services can negotiate with the different interest groups to try to get them to change their requirements or their expectations. The end result of this work is a service brief (Part 3) which defines the future external requirements that the service must meet, and their relative priority (Fig. 9.4). The remaining parts of the framework (Parts 4a, 4b, 5 and 6) are concerned with the service response — the design and delivery of the service.

Part 4a: defining the service package

The service requirements (external) are mirrored in the service specifications (internal). These are the specifications of what the service has to do to meet the requirements. At the

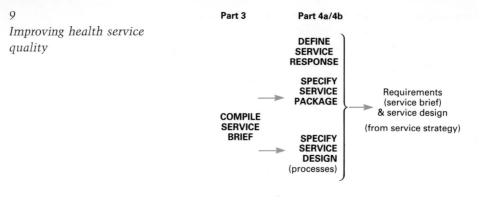

Fig. 9.4 Service brief.

broadest level this involves defining the service package.
This is what the service will offer clients (and staff) and how
the service will be provided. It is decided after considering
various service options and their practical and financial
feasibility (Chapter 2).

Once the service package is clear, this definition is put
together with the work on client-valued features to decide a
basis for differentiation. The service markets itself by differentiating itself from competitors and promoting the service
amongst referrers, potential clients and purchasers and staff.
This is the publicity link in the diagram (Fig. 9.1) that
shows how the service tells the market what it is offering.

Part 4b: service design

The service design is a more detailed specification than
the 'service package'. It specifies the overall service delivery
process, the sub-processes at different stages, and the internal
customer−supplier chains (Chapter 3). These specifications
do not need to be detailed in the early stages. They are
developed as the quality programme unfolds.

The service package and service design specifications provide the context for the daily working of the service and the
Quality Management Cycle. The specification outputs of
these steps are inputs for the next part of the framework:
the Quality Management Cycle.

There are two principles underlying this link between
service strategy and operational quality management. First,
the overall design of the service for the particular clientele
must be right before staff at the operational level can work
on improving quality. There is no point staff at this level
working at improving quality for the clients they are serving
if these are the wrong clients (e.g. not those most in need) or

the service is poorly designed to meet their needs. There are limits to the changes which they can make.

Second, staff at the operational level are not able to do market research and clarify all the external requirements of the service. But they must have information to make the quality improvements which count in the chosen market. They need to know which features of service are important to the clients and to their referrers. Staff cannot be blamed for carrying out a Quality Management Cycle which improves aspects of the service that are not important to its market position if they do not have information about what is important.

Part 5: service operation and quality management

This part of the framework (Fig. 9.5) covers the delivery and operation of the service and the Quality Management Cycle (Chapter 6). Here, the service converts the requirements and the above specifications into what staff have to do on a day-to-day basis. The service develops standards for the Client, Professional and Management Quality dimensions of the service (see specification methods in Chapter 6). The service measures performance and takes action within the Quality Management Cycle. Project teams are set up to tackle priority quality problems (Chapter 5).

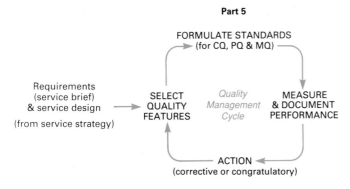

Part 5

FORMULATE STANDARDS
(for CQ, PQ & MQ)

Requirements
(service brief)
& service design

(from service strategy)

SELECT
QUALITY
FEATURES

*Quality
Management
Cycle*

MEASURE
& DOCUMENT
PERFORMANCE

ACTION
(corrective or congratulatory)

Link Quality Management Cycle to business environment

Fig. 9.5 Service operation and quality management.

Part 6: linking Quality Management Cycle to business environment

The final part of the framework is to link the Quality Management Cycle back to the service strategy. This part ensures that the service recognizes changes in the business environment, makes corresponding changes to the requirements and service brief, and feeds this back into the operational specifications in the Quality Management Cycle.

The framework therefore involves two cycles. The Quality Management Cycle for day-to-day quality control and improvement (Part 5), and a longer-term (usually annual) evaluation cycle (Part 6). The latter ensures that the specifications are linked to the business environment and requirements. Part 6 checks whether meeting specifications actually does also meet requirements, and ensures that the service brief is updated to reflect changes in requirements, and that the service design is refined.

For the sake of exposition, the framework was presented as steps for developing a new service. In practice it is usual to work with a service that is already established. In principle, the same steps are necessary to decide the future direction of the service, to market it and continually to improve quality.

Conclusion — improving health service quality

The Wel-Qual Framework links the different quality concepts and methods presented in the book and ensures that a service's quality system is related to its business strategy. The framework was developed with and for a range of health service providers and their internal service departments, to suit the particular cultural, financial and regulated 'market' circumstances of health services.

There are other frameworks which have been developed and tested more extensively in a wide range of manufacturing and service sectors, and which can be used with benefit in health services. The most well known are now commercially available as do-it-yourself packages or with consultant assistance. These are those of Deming, Juran, and Crosby (Appendix 6). Chapter 8 emphasized the importance of changing culture to any approach.

The only approach specifically for health services known at the time of writing is that of Wilson (1987). This framework was developed within the Canadian hospital system, and currently inspires some British NHS districts developing DoH-supported TQM programmes. This takes us to the first of our concluding points.

Getting started

1 *Quality requires a systematic approach.* Providers serious about introducing and pursuing a quality approach should use an established framework, or develop their own from a proven approach. This should ensure that not only do they

Quality depends on a systematic approach

Introducing quality does not mean starting from scratch, but it does mean organizing what you do within a systematic framework and using this framework to guide future action and to re-evaluate what you are doing.

Whatever approach a service uses, it should be comprehensive (involving all staff), part of everyday line management, balanced (covering Client, Professional and Management Quality dimensions), systematic and cyclical, and sustainable.

In large units, a framework should be used which will not frighten beginners, excites experts, and enthuses recalcitrant waywards (what lessons were learned introducing computers?).

It should be suitable for all, encourage continuous improvement, and make quality an integral part of the service's day-to-day work.

develop a Quality Management Cycle (Chapter 7) but that the cycle is linked to a frequently updated strategy.

Services should recognize that they already do much to assure and improve quality, and have done so for many years, although they have not called it quality action. But often what they do is piecemeal — either focusing on one aspect of the service (e.g. patient records) or on one department or profession. It is usually imbalanced and ignores one or two of the Client, Professional or Management Quality dimensions. Or it is not sustained — there is surveying and analysis but no action. There are bursts of effort and 'laurels' before the instigator leaves and things return to normal. Frequently line management and all staff are not fully involved — it is a special project.

One of the themes of the book is that the significant service improvements, cost reductions and productivity gains resulting from a quality approach, come from the mutually reinforcing effect of a number of different changes. A framework helps to achieve this, and to enable staff to take responsibility and effective action.

2 *Responsibility for quality lies first and foremost with management.* Management must aim to get everyone to take responsibility for quality, not by exhortation but by example, training in quality methods, and ensuring that time is spent applying the methods. Management must give leadership and involve staff. Staff understand the process and the problems, and can devise effective solutions with

the right training and support. If staff have come to accept poor quality at work, then it is largely the fault of management. It is the task of management to release the potential of staff to give quality service. Management can only formulate and introduce a successful quality programme to do this if they understand the quality approach and show their commitment to quality.

3 *The importance of a balance between people and processes, and between systems and relationships.* I believe the more successful quality strategies maintain such a balance. The book lays as much emphasis on the people part of the equation as on the process part. It shows how to think of the service as a process, and break it into sub-processes, how to define external and internal 'customers', and how to specify the process. But it also emphasizes the involvement of staff in this work, in measurement and in using proven quality tools and methods to improve processes.

It emphasizes relationships with clients and staff needs. The right relationships with clients are critical to avoiding dissatisfaction, and to ensuring satisfaction and high Professional Quality. A quality service must also meet the needs of staff and managers if they are to keep coming back to emotionally demanding work and to give their best. Staff cannot meet the needs of clients if their own needs are not met.

Changes in roles and relationships are as much a part of quality as effective quality tools and methods. Commitment and enthusiasm will not go far without new methods, and new structures and processes to make sure that they are applied. To make the best use of quality methods, both managers and staff have to think about their roles, responsibilities and relationships in a new way. Relationships with clients are mirrored in management−staff relationships. Changes in attitudes towards, and relationships with, clients must be paralleled by changes in internal working relationships. This is evident in the more successful community teams.

The time is right

It is easy to become despondent after reading and learning about quality and before taking the first practical steps. There seems to be such a gap between many health services as they are now and the success stories of 'quality' companies, or the 'absolute essentials' of quality, which make sense but are hard to do. There is the uncertainty about how much to invest in quality and how long it will take to produce savings or higher income. Finance is tighter than ever, morale is low, staff are shell-shocked by so many changes, and there seem to be so many other priorities.

In fact there has never been a better time to begin a serious and sustained quality strategy. Purchasers want evidence of quality and any service which introduces a quality approach will gradually achieve a competitive advantage. Staff and consumer groups are concerned about quality and see it as a way of preventing standards from falling. Any change which values staff and gives them the opportunity to contribute in an effective and meaningful way will be welcomed.

I hope this book provides a few ideas and some help to those who are concerned about the future of the NHS and to those who are rebuilding it, as well as those in other health services facing similar challenges. We never doubt the importance of health service quality when we are on the receiving end. Our lives may depend on it.

References
and
Bibliography

General

Harvey-Jones J. (1988) *Making It Happen: Reflections on Leadership*. Fontana, London

Jaques E. (1982) The method of social analysis in social change and social research. *Clinical Sociology Review*, **1**, 50–58

Kanter R.M. (1983) *The Change Masters*, Counterpoint, London

Øvretveit J. (1986) *Organisation of Community Multidisciplinary Teams*. BIOSS, Brunel University

Øvretveit J. (1987) *The Social Analytic Method for Organizational Research*. BIOSS, Brunel University

Peters T. (1987) *Thriving on Chaos*. Macmillan, London

Peters T. (1986) *Passion for Excellence*. Macmillan, London

Porter M. (1980) *Competitive Strategies: Techniques for Analysing Industries and Competition*. Free Press, New York

Rowbottom R. (1977) *Social Analysis*. Heinemann, London

Quality — general

BSI 5750 (1987) *Quality Systems Part 1: Specification for Design/Development, Production, Installation and Servicing*. British Standards Institution, Milton Keynes

Crosby P. (1979) *Quality is Free*. Mentor, New York

Crosby P. (1985) *Quality Without Tears*. Mentor, New York

Crosby P. (1986) *Quality Improvement Through Defect Prevention*. Training Package. Crosby Associates, Richmond

Deming W.E. (1986) *Out of the Crisis*. MIT, Cambridge, Mass

Feigenbaum A.V. (1963) *Total Quality Control*. McGraw-Hill, New York

Gummesson E. (1987) *Quality — The Ericsson Approach*. Ericsson, Stockholm, Sweden

Hutchins D. (1990) *In Pursuit of Quality*. Pitman, London

Ishikawa K. (1985) *What is Total Quality Control? — The Japanese Way*. Prentice Hall, Englewood Cliffs, New Jersey

Ishikawa, K., ed. (1986) *A Guide to Quality Control*. Kraus International Publications, White Plains, New York

Juran J.M. and Gryna F.M. (1980) *Quality Planning and Analysis*. McGraw-Hill, New Delhi

Juran J.M. (1964) *Managerial Breakthrough*. McGraw-Hill, New York

Juran J.M. (1988) *Juran on Planning for Quality*. Free Press, New York

Robinson R. (1984) *Quality Circles: A Practical Guide*. Gower Press, London

Schonberger R.J. (1982) *Japanese Manufacturing Techniques.* Free Press, New York

Walton M. (1986) *The Deming Management Method.* New Dodd, Putnam, New York

Service quality

Albrecht K. and Zomke R. (1985) *Service America: Doing Business in the New Economy.* Warner, New York

Albrecht K. and Bradford L. (1990) *The Service Advantage.* Dow Jones, Irwin, Illinois

Dale A. and Wooler S. (1988) *Strategy and Organization for Service.* The Programme for Service, BIOSS, Brunel University

Davidow W.H. and Uttal B. (1989) *Total Customer Service.* Harper & Row, London

Denton D.K. (1989) *Quality Service.* Gulf Publishing, London

Heskett J.L. (1986) *Managing in the Service Economy.* Harvard Business School Press

Heskett J.L., Sasser W.E. and Hart C. (1990) *Service Break-throughs.* Free Press, New York

Hopson B. and Scally M. (1989) *12 Steps to Success Through Service.* Lifeskills Publishing, Leeds

Johnston R. (1987) A framework for developing a quality strategy in a customer processing operation. *International Journal of Quality Relations Management,* **4**, 4, 37−46

Local Government Training Board (1987) *Getting Closer to the Public.* LGTB, Arndale Centre, Luton

Moores B., ed. (1986) *Are They Being Served?* Phillip Allen, London

Norman R. (1984) *Service Management: Strategy and Leadership in Service Businesses.* Wiley, London

Ong R. and Humphries P. (1990) Partners in need. *Health Services Journal,* 5th July, 1002−3

Øvretveit J. (EMI) (1988) *Improving Manufacturing Process Quality.* The Programme for Service, BIOSS, Brunel University

Øvretveit J. (1989) *The MAPS-Qual Process: A Computer Assisted Model for the USA National Quality Award.* The Programme for Service, BIOSS, Brunel University

Øvretveit J. (1989) *Business Strategy Should Drive the Quality Programme.* The Programme for Service, BIOSS, Brunel University

Parasuraman A., *et al.* (1985) A conceptual model of service quality and its implications for future research. *Journal of Marketing,* **49**, Autumn, 41−50.

Parasuraman A., *et al.* (1988) SERVQUAL: a multiple item scale for measuring consumer perceptions of service quality. *Journal of Retailing,* Spring, 12−40

Parasuraman A., *et al.* (1990) *Delivering Service Quality.* Macmillan, London

Pollitt C. (1990) Doing business in the Temple? Managers and quality assurance in the public services. *Public Administration*, **68**, 4, 435−52

TARP (1980) *Consumer Complaint Handling in America: Summary of Findings and Recommendations.* White House Office of Consumer Affairs, Washington, USA

Shostack G.L. (1984) Designing services that deliver. *Harvard Business Review*, Jan/Feb

Wyckoff D. (1984) New tools for achieving service quality. *The Cornell HRA Quarterly*, Nov, 78−91

Zeithaml V., *et al.* (1985) Problems and strategies in service marketing. *Journal of Marketing*, **49**, Spring, 33−46

Health service quality − general

Berwick D. (1989) Continuous improvement as an ideal in health care. *New England Journal of Medicine*, **320**, 1, 53−56

BMJ (1991) Oregon revises health care priorities. *British Medical Journal*, **302**, 9, 549

DoH (1989) *Working for Patients.* HMSO, London

Donabedian A. (1980) *Exploration in Quality Assessment and Monitoring Volume I. Definition of Quality and Approaches to its Assessment.* Health Administration Press, University of Michigan, Ann Arbor

High D. (1987) *Management of Quality.* Institute of Health Service Management, London

Kent P. (1991) Apologies are the best insurance. Letter. *Health Services Journal*, 21 March, 10

Kerruish A., Wickings I. and Tarrent P. (1988) Information from patients as a management tool. *Health & Hospital Service Review.* April, 64−67

Kinston W. (1988) *Making General Management Work.* BIOSS, Brunel University

Maxwell R. (1984) Quality assessment in health. *British Medical Journal*, **288**, 1470−72

McLaughlin C.P. and Kaluzny A.D. (1990) Total quality management in health: Making it work. *Health Care Management Review*, **15**, 3, 7−14

NDT (1991) *National Development Project on Quality Improvement in Health Care.* Harvard Community Health Plan, 10 Brookline Place West, Brookline, Mass 02146, USA

Øvretveit J. (1990) *Quality Health Services.* BIOSS, Brunel University

Øvretveit J. (1990) *Future Organization of NE Essex Mental Health Services.* Severalls Hospital, Colchester

Pollitt C. (1987) Capturing quality? The quality issue in British and American health policies. *Journal of Public Policy*, **7**, 71–91

Sage A. and Kingman S. (1990) Doctors drop 'unprofitable' female patients. *The Independent on Sunday*, 4th Feb, p. 3.

Shaeff R. (1991) *Marketing for Health Services*. Open University Press, Milton Keynes

Sargent J. (1991) Knowing your market. *Health Services Journal*, 14 Feb, 24–25

Wilson C. (1987) *Hospital-Wide Quality Assurance*. WB Saunders, Eastbourne

Medical and professional audit

Asbaugh D.G. and MacKean R.S. (1976) The philosophy and use of audit. *JAMA*, **236**, 1485–88

Buck N., *et al.* (1987) *Report of a Confidential Enquiry into Perioperative Deaths*. Nuffield Provincial Hospitals Trust, King's Fund, London

Dixon N. (1989) *A Guide to Medical Audit*. Conference Proceedings, National Association of Quality Assurance in Health Care, Hereford, May 1989, 29–31

DoH (1989) *Report on Confidential Enquiries into Maternal Deaths in England and Wales 1982–84*. HMSO, London

DoH (1989) *Working Paper 6 — Medical Audit*. HMSO, London

DoH (1989) *Medical Audit in the Family Practitioner Services*. HMSO, London

DoH (1991) *Medical Audit in the Hospital and Community Health Services*. HC(91)2, January, DoH, London

Essex B. and Bate J. (1991) Audit in general practice by a receptionist: a feasibility study. *British Medical Journal*, **302**, 573–6

Fowkes F.G.R., Hall R., Jones J.H., *et al.* (1986) Trail of strategy for reducing use of laboratory tests. *British Medical Journal*, **292**, 883–5

Fowkes F.G.R. and Mitchell M.W. (1985) Audit reviewed: does feedback on performance change clinical behaviour? *Journal of the Royal College of Physicians of London*, **19**, 251–4

Frater A. and Spiby J. (1990) *Measured Progress — Medical Audit for Physicians*. NW Thames Regional Health Authority, London

Gruer R., Gunn A.A., Gordon D.S. and Ruckley C.V. (1986) Audit of surgical audit. *Lancet*, **i**, 23–6

Henderson J., *et al.* (1989) Day case surgery: geographical variation, trends and readmission rates. *Journal of Epidemiology and Community Health*, **43**, 301–5

References

Heron J. (1979) *Peer Review Audit: Collected Papers*. British Postgraduate Medical Federation, University of London

Jost T. (1990) *Assuring the Quality of Medical Practice.* Kings Fund Project Paper No 82, London

Kemple T.J. and Hayter S.R. (1991) Audit of diabetes in general practice. *British Medical Journal*, **302**, 451–3

Kilty J. (1979) *Self and Peer Assessment and Peer Audit.* Human Potential Research Project, Surrey University

King's Fund Quality Assurance Programme (1989) *Medical Audit Abstracts*. King's Fund Centre, London

Marinker, M., ed. (1990) Medical Audit and General Practice. British Medical Association, London

NCEPOD (1989) *National Confidential Enquiry into Perioperative Deaths Report*. NCEPOD, London

Øvretveit J. (1988) *A Peer Review Process for Improving Service Quality.* BIOSS, Brunel University

Pearson, A., ed. (1987) *Nursing Quality Measurement: Quality Assurance Methods for Peer Review.* Wiley, London

Pendleton D., *et al.* (1986) *In Pursuit of Quality — Approaches to Performance Review in General Practice.* Royal College of General Practitioners, London

RCOG (1990) *Interim Guidelines on Medical Audit.* Royal College of Obstetricians and Gynaecologists, London

RCP (1989) *Medical Audit — A First Report. What, Why and How?* Royal College of Physicians of London

RCS (1989) *Guidelines to Clinical Audit in Surgical Practice.* Royal College of Surgeons of England, London

Rutstein D.D., Berenburg W., Chalmers T.C., *et al.* (1976) Measuring the quality of medical care: a clinical method. *New England Journal of Medicine*, **294**, 582–88

Sandeman D.R. and Cummins B.C. (1986) The provenance of extradural haematomas. *British Medical Journal*, **292**, 522–23

Sellu D.P., *et al.* (1986) Audit: its effect on the performance of a surgical unit in a DGH. *Hospital and Health Services Review*, **82**, 64–9

Shaw C. (1989) *Medical Audit: A Hospital Handbook.* King's Fund Centre, London

Young D.W. (1980) An aid to reducing unnecessary investigations. *British Medical Journal*, **281**, 1610–11

Quality assurance and accreditation

Brooks T. and Pitt C. (1990) The standard bearers. *Health Services Journal*, 30 Aug, 1286–7

BSI (1990) *Quality Management and Quality System Elements — Draft Guidelines for Services.* British Standards Institution, Milton Keynes

Dixon P. and Carr-Hill R. (1989) *The NHS and its Customers III: Consumer Feedback — A Review of Current Practice.* Centre of Health Economics, University of York

Duckett S. (1983) Changing hospitals: the role of hospital accreditation. *Social Science and Medicine*, **17**, 1573—79

Duckett S., Coombs E. and Schmiede A. (1980) *Hospital Accreditation in New South Wales.* Australian Studies in Health Services Accreditation, No. 39

Fuchs V. (1990) *Medicare's Peer Review Organizations.* Congressional Research Service, Washington

Grol R. (1990) National standards of quality of care in general practice: attitudes of general practitioners and response to a set of standards. *British Journal of General Practice*, **40**, 361—4

Kitson A.L. (1987) *Nurse Quality Assurance Directory.* Royal College of Nursing, London

Kogan M., *et al.* (1984) *Evaluation of the Management Advisory Service and Performance Review Trials.* Department of Government, Brunel University, or King's Fund Publications

Lewis C.E. (1984) Hospital accreditation. *New Zealand Hospital*, **36**, 8, 15—17

Lohr K.N., ed. (1990) *Medicare: a Strategy for Quality Assurance.* Vol. 1, Institute of Medicine/National Academy Press, Washington DC

HCFA (1988) *Medicare Hospital Mortality Information.* Government Printing Office, Washington DC

Marchment M., Morgan J. and Russel M. (1988) Introducing quality assurance to managers at unit level. *Hospital and Health Services Review*, April, 56—59

NAWCH (1987) *Quality Checklist: Caring for Children in Hospital.* National Association for the Welfare of Children in Hospital, London

NAQA (1990) *Quality in Contracts — a Collection of Papers.* National Association of Quality Assurance in Health Care, Hereford

Naym (1988) in King's Fund Quality Improvements Programme (1990) *Organizational Audit (Accreditation UK): Standards for an Acute Hospital*, King's Fund Centre, London

Pennsylvania Health Care Cost Containment Council (1989) *Hospital Effectiveness Report.* HE1—4—88, Vol. 1, Harrisburg

Roberts J.S., Coale J.G. and Redman R.R. (1987) A history of the joint commission on accreditation of hospitals. *JAMA*, **258**, 936—40

Roberts H. (1990) *Outcome and Performance in Health Care.* Public Finance Foundation, London

Rooney E.M. (1988) A proposed quality system specification

References

for the National Health service. *Quality Assurance*, **14**, 45–53

Shaw C., Hurst M. and Stone S. (1988) *Towards Good Practice in Small Hospitals: Some Suggested Guidelines*. National Association of Health Authorities, Birmingham

Sketris I. (1988) *Health Service Accreditation — An International Overview*. King's Fund Centre, London

Wilson C. (1989) *Quality Assurance*. Journal and Conference Proceedings, National Association of Quality Assurance in Health Care, Hereford

Glossary of terms

Accreditation An assessment by an external agency of an individual or organization against defined criteria.

Business strategy A vision of the position the service is to reach in the market and a five year plan of how to get there, including financial, personnel and other sub-plans, as well as a service strategy and a quality strategy. Includes a mission statement.

Client Quality Clients' views of the extent to which the service gives them what they want and expect. (The term 'client' is used instead of 'patient' to refer to the direct beneficiary of the service. 'Patient' suggests a more passive involvement than 'client', and 'client' is a more general term which also covers beneficiaries of community services. 'Customer' suggests financial exchange, and is used here as a general term.)

Client dissatisfaction The degree to which the clients' experience of the service falls short of expectations.

Client satisfaction The degree to which the clients' experience of the service exceeds their expectations, at a particular time.

Evaluation Judging the value of something by making a comparison. (Key question: is what was intended the best thing? Are there better ways of doing this?)

Indicator A measure which is used to indicate the occurrence of an event, where a direct measure cannot be used.

Level of service The amount of service provided, as represented by a service measure.

Management Quality The efficient and productive use of resources to meet customer requirements, within prescribed limits and directives. Whether the service delivery process is designed and operated to use resources in the most efficient way to meet customer requirements, without duplication, errors and waste.

Measure A quantitative representation of a subjective judgement (e.g. subjective rating), or a count of the occurrence of an event (e.g. number of deaths), or an indication of quantity on a standardized scale (e.g. waiting time, temperature, radiation levels).

Monitoring Observing activity in relation to defined specifications, standards or targets, directly or through reports or indicators. (Key question: did what was intended actually happen?)

Professional audit A systematic approach to improving Professional Quality, usually through a Quality Correction Cycle, but sometimes through a Quality Management Cycle involving a full set of Professional Quality standards for the service.

Professional Quality Professionals' judgment of the extent to which the service meets clients' needs as assessed by

163

professionals, and the extent to which professional procedures and methods are used that are believed to be necessary to meet needs. (Whether assessments and treatments are performed in the right way, and produce the required outcomes, as judged by professionals.)

Quality assurance All activities undertaken to predict and prevent poor quality. (BSI definition: 'A management system designed to give the maximum confidence that a given acceptable level of quality of service is being achieved with a minimum of total expenditure.')

Quality audit A documentation and review of a service's quality system to find out if Quality Correction Cycles and Quality Management Cycles are working to good effect.

Quality control 'The process through which we measure actual quality performance, compare it with standard and act on the difference' (Juran & Gryna 1980).

Quality Correction Cycle A series of steps for using quality methods to discover and remove the cause of a quality problem once and for all. (The aim is to improve one aspect of service quality. The steps are: definition of the problem, gathering ideas about causes, gathering data to find the causes which account for most of the problem, deciding action to remove causes, and evaluation of action.)

Quality Management Cycle A series of steps for controlling and improving all dimensions of quality using quality methods. (The steps are: selection of quality features, setting standards, measuring performance, analysing and presenting performance and deciding action (which may involve a Quality Correction Cycle)).

Quality policy A guide to action and a set of principles and philosophy which governs how people should act to improve quality.

Quality programme A 1–2-year plan for improving quality with targets and return on investment estimates.

Quality strategy A 3–5-year plan for introducing and improving service quality which supports the service and business strategy and includes a number of quality programmes.

Quality system 'The organizational structure, responsibilities, procedures, processes and resources for implementing quality management.' (BSI definition). (A quality system ensures that the service carries out quality cycles to make improvements by making sure staff have the training, responsibilities are defined, etc.)

Service Understanding another person's needs and responding in a way that meets those needs. An organization that does this for many people.

Service quality Meeting client requirements at the lowest cost to the organization, or meeting the needs of those most in need of the service at the lowest cost and within prescribed directives.

Service strategy A 3–5-year plan defining the target client group and the type of service to be provided to meet their needs.

Standard The level of performance to be achieved, as defined by a level to be achieved on a measure. This is a specific definition of a standard in terms of the level of performance to be achieved on a particular measure. If there is no measure there cannot be a standard. Other conceptions of standard include a general statement of a subject of attention or a statement of how a person should act, as in a procedure or code of ethics.

Sub-service A smaller organizational unit or a programme within a service which aims to meet the specific needs of a defined client group.

Quality audit checklist

Use: as a guide for collecting information on the quality of a service, for the purpose of:

- Providers to undertake (i) a collective staff review, (ii) to decide priorities and strategy for improving quality, or (iii) to prepare a report on quality systems and results for prospective purchasers
- Purchasers to assess the current quality status of a service

Market research, targeting and second-order Client Quality

Knowledge of customer segments and needs

1 Does the service have sufficiently reliable information to identify separate current and potential client groupings which have distinct needs and demands?

Use of knowledge for service strategy

2 Is this information used to define target population(s) and to decide priorities and objectives for each population?

Results

3 What evidence does the service hold about what the target population(s) and purchasers know about the service, and their use of the service compared to ideal use?

4 Does the service have (i) systems for ensuring that time and resources are allocated to priority customers (e.g. those who need it most), (ii) evidence of the effectiveness of these systems, and (iii) how effective are these systems?

First-order Client Quality

Information, systems, analysis and reporting

5 What information does the service collect about

(a) Customer views of the service (especially the extent to which they think it meets their needs)?

(b) How cost effective, reliable and appropriate are the systems for the service? (Systems for finding out about, and documenting dissatisfaction (complaints), and satisfaction);

(c) Does the information, analysis and presentation of this information give clear indication to staff of where and how to make improvements, and the features of service which are valued by customers?

(d) Are there quality standards and procedures which have been derived from evidence of what is most important to customers, and are they regularly reviewed in relation to recent evidence?

6 How adequate and effective are the systems for regularly informing staff and management about customers views?

Results

7 How do customers rate the service? (Do customers have usable comparisons?)

8 How adequate is staff knowledge of customer likes and dislikes?

9 What are the number, speed and effectiveness of the changes recently made to respond to customer views?

Professional Quality

10 What is the professional judgement (internal and/or external) about:
(a) The appropriateness and effectiveness of the targeting;
(b) The extent to which professionally-assessed needs are met for the customers who receive the service;
(c) The adequacy of the professional standards and procedures;
(d) The systems for monitoring and documenting that the standards and procedures are observed;
(e) The extent to which the standards and procedures are observed;
(f) The adequacy of the involvement of professional staff in planning and managing the service?

Management Quality

11 How accurate and comprehensive is the information on different cost items (especially unit costs), and is the relevant information presented and used by different staff to control costs?
12 Are there regular reports on the cost of quality (estimates of the current cost of poor quality prevention costs)?
13 Is there a process-flow analysis of the service and,
(a) Are the current key fail points and opportunities for error identified and under improvement?
(b) Do staff know their part in the overall process?
(c) Do non-direct customer contact staff know who they are serving and their 'customers' requirements?
14 Are higher management or contractor requirements clear, and to what extent does the service comply with these requirements?

Quality assurance

Structure
15 Are there staff with a specialist knowledge of and re-sponsibility for quality, and is there a satisfactory division of responsibilities between them and line managers?
Systems
16 How well does the service identify, specify, monitor and control variables which affect quality?

Documentation and penetration

17 Are there clearly described, widely understood and used quality policies, sets of programmes, reports, audits and reviews?

Human resources

Planning

18 How adequate is the human resources plan in relation to the service strategy?

Results

19 Are the numbers, skills, knowledge and experience of staff relevant to the needs of customers, and other work in the service (e.g. finance, quality techniques and systems)?

20 (a) Is each staff member clear about their responsibilities, priorities, who their manager is, their current performance, and their primary work team, and any other groups they are a member of, and,

(b) Are there systems for ensuring that staff know what is expected of them and their current performance (e.g. job descriptions, induction, performance appraisal)?

21 How do absenteeism, staff turnover, overtime, dismissals, and disciplinaries compare with similar services?

22 How adequate is training and the opportunities for career development (especially quality and multidisciplinary training)?

The Maps-Qual process for quality audit and developing strategy

Introduction

The Maps-Qual process enables a group to examine collectively the quality of their service, agree priority areas for improvement, and formulate a quality strategy. The process is based on criteria developed for the Malcum Baldridge National Quality Award, and can be used to prepare a strategy to compete successfully for the award. The process can also be used as part of a quality training and development programme. A process is also available for services to prepare for BSI 5750 registration, based on the new BSI draft for services (BSI 1990).

This appendix describes the National Quality Award, the Maps-Qual process, and the benefits of using the process. A technical document is available describing details of the process and of the computer model and software used in the process.

The Malcum Baldridge National Quality Award

The award was established in 1987 in a climate of concern about US international competitiveness. Its purpose is to promote quality awareness, recognize quality achievements of US companies, and to publicize successful quality strategies. The award was developed by the US Department of Commerce in collaboration with many quality experts and organizations. Each year two awards may be given in three categories: manufacturing organizations or subsidiaries, service organizations or subsidiaries, and small businesses. Organizations applying for the award are expected to have an excellent quality measurement system and to provide proof of quality improvements.

Assessment

The applicant organization is examined by a group of leading quality experts who judge the organization against set criteria. The emphasis is on quality achievement and improvement demonstrated by the quantitative data provided by the applicant organization.

The examination assesses what the organization is doing and has achieved in seven 'quality-producing' categories:
1 Leadership.
2 Information and analysis.
3 Strategic quality planning.
4 Human resource utilization.
5 Quality assurance of products and services.
6 Results from quality assurance of products and services.
7 Customer satisfaction.

Each category is further subdivided into subcategories of four to ten items. For example category (3) is made up of the four subcategories of: (i) Operational and strategic goals (for quality improvement); (ii) Planning function (describing the function and how the organization is structured to highlight quality improvement planning); (iii) Planning for quality improvement (specific plans for quality improvement), and (iv) Unique and innovative planning (any unique techniques being used for planning).

Examiners score each of these subcategories against specified criteria. For example the criteria for assessing (iv) (Unique and innovative planning) are: (a) the effectiveness of the techniques, and (b) their overall effect on the planning process. The applicant organization is expected to provide evidence which is relevant to these criteria. Finalists undergo site visits by the examiners.

Benefits of improving quality

The award categories were chosen by quality experts as being critical for achieving quality improvements. Any organization applying for the award would clearly need to review extensively its quality systems and strategy, and would benefit from such a review. Even if an organization were not to apply, the award guidelines provide a practical focus for an organization wishing to improve quality. The link between quality, profitability and market share is now widely recognized.

The Maps-Qual process

The Model for Assessing Priorities in Service Quality (Maps-Qual) is a computer model based on the National Quality Award categories and criteria. The Maps-Qual process enables a group to use these criteria to decide the most important areas to focus on in order to make the greatest improvement in quality, given their current quality performance. The group usually includes senior managers and quality specialists with the power to make significant changes, and who wish to review their quality performance and decide a quality improvement strategy.

The steps of the process involve:

1 Identification of group members to take part in the process, and preparation for the process workshop usually lasting 2–3 days.

2 At the start of the workshop the process workshop facilitator explains the categories and subcategories in the National Quality Award and included in Maps-Qual. The group familiarize themselves with the categories and their

meaning for their organization, and delete criteria which are not relevant.

3 The group considers each subcategory and its assessment criteria in turn, and discuss current organizational performance, with the emphasis on evidence of performance. The group agrees a current provable performance score for the subcategory (out of 100%), in comparison to a possible ideal (or competitors).

4 After scoring performance on all subcategories, the model computes the rank order of priority of the subcategories. That is, it indicates which subcategories the group needs to focus time and effort on improving, and which areas will have a minimal impact on overall quality performance. (The computer takes the group's assessment of current performance, and using the weightings of importance of each subcategory set by the award guidelines, it calculates which subcategories rank highest in terms of low performance but high weighting).

5 The group formulates a strategy and timetable for improving quality performance, guided by the computer listings, and by further computer analysis of the categories (The Maps-Qual Technical Document gives details of sensitivity analyses and other ways of exploring the model to aid decision-making).

Outcomes from using the process

The model and process are not just to help organizations compete more successfully for the National Quality Award, but are intended to help any organization to review and improve quality. Amongst the benefits of the process are:

1 Training in quality: participants learn to apply the award categories to their own organization and learn the relative importance of each category in its impact on quality, as assessed by the award, and as judged by themselves. This is particularly important for general managers who may only have a general knowledge of quality issues.

2 Developmental: key individuals with a potential impact on quality come together in a group and, through the process, form a common understanding of what quality means in their organization, what affects quality, and how the organization currently performs. Most importantly, they agree the key areas for improvement with a thorough understanding of the reasons for making changes. The process is a powerful team-building method which confronts and works through conflicting views.

3 Focuses effort: the model enables the group to assess quickly priority areas for improvement, and to understand the effects of making improvements in different areas on

overall quality. Often it is the more costly changes which in fact prove to have little impact on quality relative to other changes.

More information on the process and about on-site workshops to audit a service and develop strategy is available from Dr J. Øvretveit, Health Services Centre, Brunel University, Uxbridge, Middx. (Tel. 0895 56461).

Introduction

The purpose of this questionnaire is to help your department identify your internal (and external) customers and suppliers, to assess your own and your suppliers' performance in giving service, and to help your department to agree the service improvements to be made.

The questionnaire asks you to (i) say who you think your customers are (the internal departments or external customers to whom you provide a service), (ii) say who your main suppliers are.

We will compare your ideas about who your customers are with other departments' views about whether you are a key supplier to them. The questionnaire then asks you (iii) to guess what you think are the important features of service for your customers, and (iv) how well you think you are meeting these customer requirements. We will compare this with what your customers actually say.

The information from the questionnaires will be used in feedback and service improvement workshops to clarify your customers' requirements and to consider the changes which you need to make to improve your service to them.

We recommend that you involve staff in your department in formulating answers to the questionnaire, by for example, going through the questions in a departmental meeting (estimated time 1−2 hours).

Name: Department:

Job title:

Staff involved in completing the questionnaire:

A Identifying customers and priorities

1 *Your department's customers*
Focusing on the services provided by your department, who are the immediate internal (and/or external) 'customers' for your product?

2 *Priorities between your immediate customers*
If one of your department's immediate customers gets priority service, mark this customer with a 'P1' in your list above. Of all the other customers, do any get priority? If so mark this one (or two etc.) with a 'P2'. Then mark others according to priority treatment (P3, P4, etc.).

3 *Identifying suppliers to your department*
Who supplies your department with services? (i.e. for whom

are you a 'customer'). List the main internal as well as external suppliers on whom you rely in order that you can produce your service and product.

4 *Who is your most important supplier?*
(Using your and others answers to these questions we can find out if suppliers and customers agree or disagree about their relationship.)

B Evaluating your suppliers' performance

5 *Your view of your suppliers' performance*
What are the *features* of your suppliers' services which are most important to you (e.g. lowest price, correct delivery reliable product, etc.). Please explain these clearly so that we can understand what you mean.

List these first, and then put them in rank order of importance by putting '1' next to the feature which you think is the most important, and '2' next to the second most important, and so on.

Feature of supplier's service	Rank order of importance	Rating (see Question 6)
....	....	....
....	....	....
....	....	....

6 *Do your suppliers always meet your requirements — could they improve?*
Make a judgement of your suppliers' performance by taking your first feature, and rating their performance out of 100%. If you think that they think that they fully meet your requirements, give a rating of 100%. Rate all the features you listed above.

7 *Give some suggestions for your suppliers as to what they could do to improve their service to you.*

8 *What do you think prevents your suppliers from giving you a better service?*

C Evaluating your service performance

9 *From your immediate customers' point of view (that is, those you listed in Question 1), what are the features of service which you think are most important to them? (e.g. lowest price, correct delivery, reliable product, etc.)*
Please explain these clearly so that we can understand what you mean.

174

List these first, and then put them in rank order of importance by putting '1' next to the feature which you think that they think is the most important, and '2' next to the second most important (from their point of view), and so on.

Feature of our service from our customers point of view	Rank order of importance	Rating (see Question 10)
. . . .	. . . .	. . . .
. . . .	. . . .	. . . .
. . . .	. . . .	. . . .

10 *Your customers' view of your performance*
How well do you think you meet customer requirements on each feature? Make a judgement of your customers' view of your performance by taking your first feature, and rating your performance out of 100%, from the customer's point of view. (If you think that they think that you fully meet their requirements, give a rating of 100%.) Rate all the features you listed above.

11 *List some things that you could do to improve your service to your customers*

Thank you for working at this questionnaire. We will discuss the results with you when we have analysed the responses.

The peer review process

The process follows a sequence of steps, each of which builds on the steps before, and which aim to develop and apply staff skills to evaluate and improve their service.

The first 2-day peer review workshop starts with each person considering their own work with each of their clients, and using this as a basis to think about their collective service aims, and about the standards of quality of the service. Staff then discuss and agree what they think their service aims and standards should be. Staff then do a rough rating of their own collective service, noting where they do and do not have evidence about their performance in relation to each of their agreed aims and quality standards. They then consider what changes they think they would need to make to improve their ratings, and set these changes as target improvements for the next 3 months. Finally they consider what evidence they would need to collect in the future to give themselves routine and objective feedback about their performance in relation to their aims and standards.

Day 2 of the workshop starts with staff presenting their self-assessment to staff from a similar service (service 'B') by listing their aims and standards, by giving their rough assessment of their performance, stating their targets for improvements, and by saying how they propose to gain evidence about their performance in the future. The visiting staff group then changes place and presents their service: they outline their aims and standards and their assessment of their service and invite questions.

The two groups then separately work out the feedback which they will give about their peer's presentation, and meet together to exchange feedback. Each group then uses their peer's comments and ideas to revise their own quality review package. They revise their aims and standards, decide the information they need to collect and the methods to use, as well as the target improvements which they will make.

Over the next 3 months, and before the second review workshop, each group sets up the routine information gathering and recording systems which they decided, gather any special information which was thought important, and works towards target improvements. In addition clients, referrers and other relevant parties prepare to give staff their views about the service strengths and weaknesses.

The second workshop starts with service groups exchanging reports as before. Each group presents:
- Their more accurate self-evaluation, in the light of the evidence which they have gathered
- Progress on the target improvements which were decided at the last workshop
- Ideas about a system for routine feedback about their

performance, and about a routine review process
The groups comment on and discuss each other's reports.

On the second day of this workshop, clients, referrers and others give each group their assessment of the service, and staff alter their aims and standards to better reflect client views and needs. Finally each group and their manager plans and decides the new target improvements, and the details of the information system and routine quality review procedure which they will use in the future.

More details are provided in the report, Øvretveit (1988).

Quality
frameworks —
key points

Juran's 10 steps to quality improvement (Juran 1988)

1 Build awareness of the need and opportunity for improvement
2 Set goals for improvement
3 Organize to reach the goals (establish a quality council, identify problems, select projects, appoint teams, designate facilitators)
4 Provide training
5 Carry out projects to solve problems
6 Report progress
7 Give recognition
8 Communicate results
9 Keep score
10 Maintain momentum by making annual improvement part of the regular systems and processes of the company

Crosby's 14-step quality improvement programme

Crosby's 14-step quality improvement programme (Crosby 1979) is one of the most practical guides for a major change in larger units, but the general approach is also relevant to a small unit. The following is a brief summary:

1 Management commitment: ensuring management are committed to the programme
2 Quality improvement teams: Representatives from each department, orientated to the purpose of the team
3 Quality measurement: Establishing measures of quality in each area
4 Cost of quality evaluation: By accounts department to find out where corrective action will save the most
5 Quality awareness: Sharing with employees the cost of poor quality and raising awareness of where these costs come from
6 Corrective action: Supervisors work with staff to eliminate poor quality
7 Ad hoc committee for the zero defects programme: Investigates the Zero Defects Concept and suggests a programme
8 Supervisor training: All managers understand the programme and their role
9 Zero defects day: Establish zero defects as the performance standard for the company on one day
10 Goal setting: Following the day, setting clear quality goals in each work group
11 Error cause removal: A one-page form for each employee to describe any problem which prevents them from performing error-free work. Information passed to appropriate group, who reply to the problem

12 Recognition: Award programmes

13 Quality councils: Quality specialists and quality team leaders meet to decide how to solve quality problems and upgrade the programme

14 Do it over again: Set up new quality group, and follow through the steps again

Deming's 14 points for management (Deming 1986)

1 Create constancy of purpose toward improvement of product and service

2 Adopt the new philosophy. We can no longer live with commonly accepted levels of delay, mistakes, defective materials, and defective workmanship

3 Cease dependence on mass inspection. Require, instead, statistical evidence that quality is built in

4 End the practice of awarding business on the basis of price tag

5 Find problems. It is management's job to work continually on the system

6 Institute modern methods of training on the job

7 Institute modern methods of supervision of production workers. The responsibility of foremen must be changed from numbers to quality

8 Drive out fear, so that everyone may work effectively for the company

9 Break down barriers between departments

10 Eliminate numerical goals, posters, and slogans for the workforce asking for new levels of productivity without providing methods

11 Eliminate work standards that prescribe numerical quotas

12 Remove barriers that stand between the hourly worker and his right to pride of workmanship

13 Institute a vigorous programme of education and training

14 Create a structure in top management that will push every day on the above 13 points

Postscript: reflections of a researcher-patient

Two weeks after finishing this book I had an unexpected opportunity to carry out participant research into the subject in a UK hospital. I was an in-patient for 4 days and underwent an operation for a fractured elbow. Determined to turn the experience to some useful end, I decided to record and analyse my experience as a patient. The following outlines some of my reflections on health service quality after being on the receiving end. It illustrates and comments on some of the quality concepts described.

One useful method proved to be the simple framework for analysing a patient's perception of the service (Chapter 3), which I had previously used with staff groups. As soon as I recovered from anaesthesia I acquired a note pad and used this framework to record my 'career' through the service, from registering at Accident and Emergency at 8.30 p.m. on the Wednesday night to leaving the ward at 6.00 p.m. on the Saturday night. Using this framework brought home the importance of systematic and objective methods to diagnose quality issues. One reason is subjective bias. At the time I had no complaints and would have rated myself as 'satisfied' with the service. But after looking over my notes I became more aware that there were things which I was not happy with, and a number of avoidable quality problems.

Another reason is that the framework helped to locate and identify the different quality problems and to assess their relative importance. Using the framework I could read off the list of problems, and the departments/professions which appeared to be the source of the problem. Looking over my notes, the weak link in the chain was undoubtedly X-ray, in terms of the related quality problems of waiting time and error rate.

My immediate post-operation X-ray was of such poor quality that I had to be taken back (awake this time, and without painkillers) for another. I waited at least an hour in a wheelchair in a queue in a cold corridor, naked apart from pants, a blanket and a bandaged arm, hoping that the new X-ray technician would keep my 'ticket' in order in the list. Part of the delay was that the patient two places before me was called back three times before they got it right.

This experience also highlighted how groups affect individual's perceptions. The X-ray queue was one unhappy group. Being aware of other people's frustrations allowed me to become aware of my own discomforts which I had largely ignored in the Dunkirk spirit of the ward. There the hard work and cheerful attitude of the obviously short-staffed nursing team made it very difficult to be dissatisfied — how could anyone be critical of the nursing staff, given the conditions?

This latter point also reinforced the relevance of distinctions between different ways in which people perceive a health service: in terms of what they want (an ideal), what they expect (what is likely), what they think they need, what they experience at different times, and their overall impression. In each case people use a different yardstick to clarify their perception, and questionnaires may or may not indicate which yardstick to use.

It was clear that on the ward most patients' satisfaction was largely influenced by our idea of what it would be reasonable to expect of hard-pressed nursing staff. We could see others worse off and readjusted our demands. We expected little and were not dissatisfied. It would be easy for service providers to conclude that we were satisfied. But if we were judging the service against an ideal, then it left much to be desired. The situation was different in a number of respects in the X-ray queue. This was not a stable group with nurses working at sustaining a group culture, and where people were much more time-conscious.

My experience confirmed the importance of assessing both dissatisfaction (e.g. complaints) and satisfaction. On reflection my main dissatisfactions in order of priority were: poor pain control, X-ray delay and error, lack of medical information, medical arrogance, multiple doctors (I saw 8 doctors at different times (not including students)), inconsistent and contradictory information, and the bedside paper-seller ignoring my shouts and walking off with my only change for the telephone.

If I had not had these dissatisfactions, however, I would not necessarily have been satisfied — not because I'm an awkward character, but because satisfaction is a different dimension. To be satisfied I would have needed better than school-dinner food (e.g. with the choice of sugar or not in my porridge), not to have been washed a few hours after the operation when the pain was at its height, and not to be woken up with a shock at 3 a.m. by feeling antibiotics injected into my arm.

Having said this it is interesting that I still feel guilty about raising any complaint about my treatment and feel profoundly grateful to all the staff. It is almost as if the gratitude factor and low expectations made us as patients immune to noticing poor service, and any dissatisfaction would have to be great to bring us to complain. One problem is the informal and formal response to complaints, which is first to make light, then deny. It is easy to see how these conditions needlessly generate and escalate negligence claims.

My experiences affirmed two final and related points about patients' perceptions. First, that dissatisfactions and satisfactions are hierarchical and similar to a hierarchy of needs. Second, that features of service quality have different weights of importance at different times. For 12 hours after waking up after the operation, the ony thing of any importance to me was to reduce the pain. Only after the pain subsided did I become aware of other things and my attention turned to food, and then to other matters.

My main complaint was lack of pain control and it seemed at the time that both medical and nursing staff did not take this seriously. Although I was aware that they felt it risky to give any more painkillers, one doctor said that they could change the prescription, but the nurses refused to do so when I asked. Later I was told I could have more painkillers in an hour, only to be refused when the time came. I made it through to the morning ward round and was assured by the consultant that they could and would do something about the pain. I realized as I was being wheeled off to X-ray 3 hours later that nothing was going to be done.

Most of the things I have described are one patient's perceptions, recorded and structured through the use of some quality concepts. My experience also affirmed from another prospective the validity of the distinction between three dimensions of health service quality: Client Quality, Professional Quality and Management Quality. I was and still am unable to assess the Professional Quality of the service which I received, not least because I was not conscious in theatre during the most important part. (Later in the wait to be collected from X-ray I sneaked a look because I was curious to see what had been done. I saw two steel pins supporting the bone but I could not tell if it was a good job). Neither am I able to judge the Management Quality of the service, although there were signs of waste, poor organization and poor communications, especially between professions and departments.

Some of the conflicts between these different dimensions of service quality were apparent, as well as methods for resolving the conflicts. For example, to improve the Client Quality of the service I received would have meant reducing the pain, but this (as far as I know) would have conflicted with Professional Quality (the risks of more painkillers for a 'small chap'). Again, I would have been more satisfied if I had been allowed to go home a day earlier, but this would have conflicted with Professional Quality. In these instances the resolutions to the conflict were in the relationship between patient and professional staff. More discussion between us about pain control would probably have removed my dissatisfactions. I know that my rising dissatisfaction about being kept in unnecessarily was turned to respect and satisfaction by an equal exchange with the registrar. She was honest with me and said she could not keep me in against my will but they wanted to be absolutely sure that there was no infection. I was honest with her and said I did not want to cause trouble. We struck a deal whereby I could keep track of temperature and come in if the trend went up. But I knew that this happened because I had acquired power — by then I was lucid and mobile and was prepared to walk out anyway.

It was clear that the quality problems of which I became aware were not due to indifference or laziness, but that given the right conceptual tools and the time to use them there would be no difficulty in substantially raising the quality of the service. On reflection I think probably the most important factor in improving quality would be a genuine and multidisciplinary/multidepartmental desire to identify the shortcomings and really do something about them. Only then would staff begin to use and realize the power of the new quality methods. At present the biggest barrier is probably a quite understandable defensiveness and denial of being the source of quality problems, even unknowingly. I think this is partly due to staff not feeling valued.

Index